T0205589

A Computational View of Autism

Uttama Lahiri

A Computational View of Autism

Using Virtual Reality Technologies
in Autism Intervention

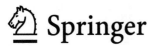 Springer

Uttama Lahiri
Department of Electrical Engineering
IIT Gandhinagar
Gujarat, India

ISBN 978-3-030-40239-6   ISBN 978-3-030-40237-2   (eBook)
https://doi.org/10.1007/978-3-030-40237-2

This Springer imprint is published by the registered company Springer Nature Switzerland AG.
The registered company address is: Gewerbestrasse 11, 6330 Cham, Switzerland

This book is dedicated to my parents,
Sri Arijit Lahiri and Smt Maya Lahiri

Preface

I was giving a lecture on 'Experimental Techniques in Cognitive Science', and after hearing about applications, the term 'autism' came up and has popped up into my mind time and again. I have been applying technical knowledge to autism-related research for almost a decade. Some students asked me, 'What is autism?' while others seem to have some idea about the topic. I usually respond by briefly explaining the genesis of the term 'autism'. Then the next question that obviously comes up is, 'What does Experimental Techniques in Cognitive Science have to do with it?' Some students know that conventional observation-based techniques are used for autism intervention. Some are aware of the term 'affective computing'. But most are unaware of the underlying relation between the conventional intervention techniques and technology that can be used for autism intervention.

This class has students from diverse educational backgrounds, including engineering, psychology, and medicine. I have tried to formulate my responses in ways that offer pertinent information to all the students, in spite of their various backgrounds.

Again, I feel like sharing my experiences when I meet families who have children with autism. While speaking to them, often it becomes apparent that in many cases they are unaware of the various assessment tools that can help to screen their child. This is necessary since, once diagnosed, these children can be referred for intervention, and early intervention has huge potential in addressing the core deficit areas characterizing these children. In spite of being educated, oftentimes I find these parents unaware of the different technological innovations that can enable them to offer such services even in their homes along with therapist-assisted intervention services.

Although research in the area of autism has progressed to a considerable extent, there are still very few books that communicate the various research findings to the different stakeholders, including students and caregivers of these children. This inspired me to present my knowledge and understanding of the applications in the area of autism research. Additionally, with my years of experience in applying computing in the area of autism research and my close involvement with special needs schools and intervention service centres for individuals with autism, I thought of presenting a blend of the different techniques in such a book, including using conventional intervention techniques and technical solutions, such as robots and computers in autism intervention. This was my motivation for writing this book.

Thus, I begin the book with the genesis of the term 'autism'. Also, I explain why it is important to be aware of this term and its prevalence, and I discuss some of the standard techniques used to assess autism. Then I present glimpses of conventional observation-based techniques for autism intervention in different educational settings. I explain the advantages and limitations in the Indian context. Then I introduce the reader to technology-based solutions using robots and computers, which can serve as complementary tools in the hands of the interventionists. While discussing computer-based applications, I offer a detailed account of the different approaches such as virtual reality, augmented reality, and others that have been deployed in the area of autism research. Based on my years of experience working in the area of virtual reality while applying it in the domain of autism-related research, I show the readers how it can be used to address some of the core deficits that characterize autism.

In short, the readers of this book can get a good idea about autism, the genesis of the term 'autism', some of the core attributes that characterize individuals who experience autism, assessment tools, and how to use technology to address at least some of the core deficits that these people face. While writing on these topics, I have tried to cite real-life examples from my own experience working with autistic children for several years in different parts of the world. Thus, this book can be informative for students, researchers, and caregivers. Also this book can serve to increase awareness about autism in society.

I am thankful to my students who put forward questions to me regarding the technologies that can serve as complementary tools (in the hands of clinicians involved in autism intervention and the families of autistic children), and I have tried to formulate my responses to them. In this process, I felt like jotting down my thoughts and presenting my understanding and knowledge to my students in the form of a book. This is how this book came about. It took me about six months to knit the contents into the form of a book.

Being an engineer by profession, and having worked with robots and computer-based platforms, namely Virtual Reality applied to autism-related research, a major part of this book is devoted to the use of such techniques in autism intervention. Apart from viewing these techniques from the user's perspective, I have tried to describe specific applications related to social communication, emotion recognition, and joint attention while presenting some of the Virtual Reality-based design considerations that might be relevant for designers developing such platforms.

Finally, I end the book with a philosophical note by bringing in the argument between Virtual Reality and reality and discussing the steps that can be taken to reduce the difference with the ultimate aim of offering a place where both typically developing individuals and individuals with autism can co-exist in a meaningful manner.

Gujarat, India   Uttama Lahiri
December 2019

Contents

Chapter 1
Autism and Its Prevalence

1.1 Genesis of the Term 'Autism'

In 1943, the term 'autism' was coined by the Austrian-American psychiatrist, physician, and social activist Leo Kanner. Kanner's published work *Autistic Disturbances of Affective Contact* presents facts and observations of eleven children with autism (Kanner 1943). He reported that these children are very intelligent, and they exhibited a desire for loneliness.

1.2 What Is Autism?

Autism is a neurodevelopmental disorder characterized by impairments in socialization and communication. This is a spectrum disorder in which every child is unique, and thus the term autism spectrum disorder (ASD) is used in many places. Individuals with autism often demonstrate difficulties in social judgment, such as deciding on appropriate social behaviours (Baron-Cohen et al. 1999; Carpenter et al. 2002). Deficits in their ability to appropriately reciprocate and in turn carry out lucid social interaction can have adverse cascading effects. Such a deficit often deters them from initiating and maintaining conversation with social partners that in turn can adversely affect their ability to develop friendships (Cai et al. 2013). Though some of the individuals with autism have a desire to make friends and build relationships, yet they struggle to start and maintain these relationships. These individuals are often characterized by their inability to understand the intention of a communicator. Specifically, in many occasions, they interpret comments from a communicator in the literal sense. They often struggle to understand the meanings of phrases such as 'tighten your belts' that they often take literally and fail to understand the inherent meaning that is one need to be cautious with spending money. Also, these individuals express eagerness to speak on their own interests without paying any attention

© Springer Nature Switzerland AG 2020
U. Lahiri, *A Computational View of Autism*,
https://doi.org/10.1007/978-3-030-40237-2_1

to the listeners' responses, often making comments that are not context relevant. As a consequence, they often appear to demonstrate out-of-context behaviour that might steal away the lucidity in the flow of thoughts during social communication with a partner.

The impairments in socialization are also related to difficulty in making eye contact with social partners (Jones et al. 2008). This is considered as one of the first symptomatic manifestations of autism. For example, while communicating with social partners, they often tend to avoid the eye region and look towards other regions of the face such as the mouth region. While eyes are considered a window into one's mind, these individuals exhibit deficits in reading other's mind that is often very important in carrying out lucid social communication. Given the fact that individuals often use different ways to express emotions, the eye region plays an important role. In many situations, the atypical looking pattern of the individuals with autism can cause them to miss some of the emotional expressions displayed by the social partner such as shrinking of the eyebrows to indicate frustration, squinting of eyes to indicate anger, etc. adversely affecting their social communication. Again, children with autism often show disengagement towards social stimuli (McGee et al. 1997; Sigman and Ruskin 1999) while demonstrating an atypical looking pattern. Specifically, their atypical viewing patterns can be attributed in part by greater fixation towards non-social objects than faces of social communicators. For example, let us consider a situation in which an interventionist (clinician) is trying to teach a child the skill of turn-taking while participating in a play in a room having various objects. The child exhibits an atypical looking pattern in which the child tends to avoid the face region of the clinician and instead focuses on different inanimate objects such as toys kept in the room. In such a scenario, if the clinician prompts the child to pick up a particular toy item by looking towards the toy, the child being preoccupied with the toys often tends to miss the prompt. A typical looking pattern often causes them to miss non-verbal cues such as body language and facial expressions of a social communicator (Moore 2002). To understand the social communication vulnerabilities of individuals with autism, research has examined how they process salient social cues, specifically from the faces of social communicators (Rutherford and Towns 2008; Jones et al. 2008). This is because appropriate reciprocation during social interaction can be facilitated if the communicators are capable of deriving socially relevant information from each other's face (Trepagnier et al. 2002). An early deficit in such a capability can contribute in part to the developmental cascade associated with core vulnerabilities of the disorder (Dawson 2008). These deficits create barriers for individuals with ASD in successful participation in community life at later stages leading to social isolation.

Added to the communication-related deficits, these individuals have restricted adaptability to variations. This is often manifested in terms of their deficit in adapting to changes in routine. For example, let us consider a child with autism is habituated to a particular routine while going to school each morning. If on a particular day, the situation at his house is such that it demands him to modify his routine so as to adjust to the situation, then the child with autism will experience severe difficulties in adapting to the change in routine. Again, the child can experience difficulties in generalizing information relevant for different situations. By generalization, I mean the process by which skills learnt in one situation can be applied to another situation. For example, let us consider two scenarios such as a bus station and a restaurant. A teacher is trying to teach a child with autism the art of occupying a seat in the passenger waiting bay area of a bus station. In this, the teacher is trying to provide the tips on how to navigate between the rows of seats and exhibit social etiquettes while occupying a seat. Such as the teacher might say to the child that if you see few chairs being empty in a particular area of the waiting bay and someone is occupying one of the chairs in that area, then it would be preferred that you do not occupy the chair that is adjacent to the chair being occupied since the adjacent seat might be meant for someone known to the individual already occupying one of the chairs. Now let us consider a restaurant environment during a busy hour in which all the tables are mostly occupied except one of the tables that is partially occupied. Post the training in a bus station scenario, the child with autism can be expected to exhibit similar behaviour in the restaurant scenario. However, the child might face difficulties in generalizing the skills learnt from the bus station scenario to the restaurant environment.

1.3   Prevalence of Autism and Awareness of It

With a prevalence rate of 1 in 150 in India (The Times of India April 5, 2012), 1 in 59 in the United States (CDC 2018) and 1 in 100 in the United Kingdom (National Statistics Survey 2012), creating effective intervention services for addressing the skill deficits characterizing autism can be considered as a pressing clinical and public health issue. Autism is four times more likely to appear in boys than in girls. In an Indian context, the prevalence of autism can be considered to be largely affected by (a) a general lack of awareness of the autism condition and (b) unwillingness of parents to accept that their child has autism. In India, such conditions are often perceived as a taboo. Additionally, a major segment of the population being rural, the awareness of such (autism) condition is limited. As a result, the condition of autism is often mistaken with other conditions. This often leads to a delay in the child getting to avail intervention services. Also, in India, such intervention services can be availed in specialized pockets such as specialized inclusive schools that are mostly situated within the urban community. In many cases, such schools are privately owned and set up by a consortium of parents having children with autism. Additionally, the cost of such intervention services is very high. Specifically, such services are often expensive, since in many cases, these demand one-on-one services with the therapist or the interventionist. Given the high cost, most have restricted accessibility to such specialized services.

1.4   How Is Autism Assessed?

Autism is often characterized by deficits in building social connections and initiating and maintaining social communication and atypical disposition in terms of interests (Ozonoff et al. 2005). Development of social linkages becomes disrupted by their atypical presence in terms of preoccupation in oneself with a limited desire to share enjoyment with others. Deficit in social communication is often manifested in terms of delay in language acquisition and development of spoken language. As far as atypical disposition is concerned, these individuals often use repetitive language, demonstrate inability to imitate and participate in pretend play and exhibit unusual adherence to routines, stereotyped body movements, unusual preoccupation with parts of objects, etc. (APA 2000).

Though these deficits are often quite visible, yet, there needs to be metrics by which one can get quantitative estimates to assess the extent of the disorder. Some of the widely used metrics are Social Responsiveness Scale (SRS), Social Communication Questionnaire (SCQ), Autism Diagnostic Observation Scheduled—Generic (ADOS-G), Autism Diagnostic Interview—Revised (ADI-R), and Childhood Autism Rating Scale (CARS).

1.4.1   Social Responsiveness Scale (SRS)

This scale seeks to get caregiver's feedback to quantify the severity of autism-related symptoms (Constantino et al. 2003). Generally, it takes about 15 min to administer this test. This scale can measure the social ability of children aged between 4 and 18 years. Again, there is a second edition of SRS that can be applicable for children aged 2.5 years through adulthood. Research has shown that the SRS has good psychometric properties and cross-cultural validity of the assessment of autism (Bölte et al. 2008, 2011). This is in the form of a questionnaire having 65 questions on topics such as social awareness, social information processing, capacity for reciprocal social communication, social anxiety or avoidance, and autistic preoccupations and traits. Each response is rated using a 4-point scale ranging from 'Not True' to 'Almost Always True'. The results obtained from the SRS are in terms of T-score with an emphasis on receptive, expressive, and motivational aspects of social behaviour and autistic preoccupations. According to Constantino (2002), the various cut-offs to the T-score are as follows:

T-score $\leq$ 59 T: This is considered as normal that is typically developing.

60 T $\leq$ T-score $\leq$ 75 T: This is considered to lie in the mild to moderate range of autism.

T- score $\geq$ 76 T: This is considered to be severe autism.

1.4.2   Social Communication Questionnaire (SCQ)

This scale is similar to the SRS in terms of being a parent report. The SCQ has a list of 40 questions with binary response options, namely 'yes' or 'no'. There are two versions of this questionnaire namely, Lifetime and Current. This is meant to be filled in by the caregivers who are aware of the developmental details and behaviour of the individual being studied. The Lifetime version offers a score that can be analysed with respect to cut-off. Generally, a cut-off score of 15 is considered. An individual getting a score greater than 15 is considered to have autism. This scale examines the child's disposition since the last 3 months. This can inform the clinician about the child's recent experiences who in turn can suggest appropriate educational plans. Some of the questions of SCQ have been adapted from the Autism Diagnostic Interview (ADI) (Rutter et al. 2003b). These questions are used to assess one on autism symptoms related to reciprocal social interaction, communication, and repetitive and stereotyped patterns of behaviour. The SCQ score can be used to discriminate ASD from non-ASD, autism vs. mental retardation, and autism vs. other aspects of ASD. The SCQ can be used to assess children aged older than 4 years, but with a mental age of at least 2 years. The mental age is different from the chronological age. The mental age can be related to an individual's intelligence. Specifically, this considers an individual having a specific age and how he or she can perform intellectually compared to one that can be performed at his or her actual age (i.e. the chronological age). While working with children with autism, the interventionists often refer to the child's mental age added to the chronological age since these children often demonstrate low mental age, particularly with respect to cognitive functioning (Hinnebusch et al. 2017).

1.4.3   Autism Diagnostic Observation Schedule: Generic (ADOS-G)

This scale is a semi-structured assessment that uses observation-based techniques. This is used to judge one on aspects such as play, social interaction, and communicative skills that in turn can be employed for identifying the presence of autism (Lord et al. 2000). This test consists of four modules (module 1, module 2, module 3, and module 4) with each module requiring observation-based evaluation for about 30 min. Only one module is administered at any given time. Each module is applicable for children and adults with different levels of development and language usage that can range from no expressive or receptive use of words to use of fluent language while expressing oneself. The therapist generally chooses a module that best matches with the expressive language skill level of the child while evaluating the social and communicative abilities of the child. The modules 1 and 2 are generally carried out while moving inside a room and evaluating the interests and level of activity of a young child or a child having very limited usage of language.

The module 1 is used for children who do not make use of spontaneous speech. This module consists of ten activities. The module 2 is used for children who have some speech, but who do not have fluency of speech. This module consists of 14 activities. The modules 3 and 4 are generally carried out while sitting at a table along with the conversation and the use of language. The module 3 is meant for individuals who are verbally fluent and demonstrate age-appropriate behaviour while playing with toys. This module consists of 13 activities. The module 4 is meant for adults who are verbally fluent and not interested in playing with toys. This module consists of 10–15 activities. Each module is used to rate an individual in language and communication, reciprocal social interaction, play or imagination or creativity, stereotyped behaviours and restricted interests, and other abnormal behaviours. A score $\geq$ 7 on communication and reciprocal social interaction indicates ASD. However, a score of $\geq$10 is considered as autistic disorder.

1.4.4 Autism Diagnostic Interview-Revised (ADI-R)

This scale seeks to obtain caregiver's views and is administered using a semi-structured interview. The scale contains 93 items. This can be used to distinguish autism from other pervasive developmental disorders (Rutter et al. 2003a). Also, ADI-R can discriminate autism from non-autism. This scale can be applied to individuals with mental age $\geq$ 18 months (Lord et al. 1997). This scale considers different aspects such as background and history, early development, acquisition and loss of skills, language and communication, social development and play, favourite activities, interests, and behaviours. Also, this is used to evaluate where each individual lies on the spectrum in terms of social reciprocity, language and communication, and restricted and repetitive activities. Specifically, this scale evaluates an individual in three domains. The first one is the social communication domain. This domain evaluates one's social interaction and communication such as whether the child demonstrates social smiling and responds to other children, can offer and seek comfort, etc. The second domain examines the restrictive or repetitive behaviour. This evaluates one in terms of having an unusual preoccupation with an object of interest, hand and finger manners, unusual sensory interest, etc. The third domain evaluates one's imitation, gesture and play, or reciprocal and peer interaction. For example, this looks at whether a child can make social use of language while interacting with peers. A cut-off score of 22 on reciprocal social interaction, communication, restricted and repetitive patterns of behaviour, and evidence of abnormal development before the age of 36 months indicates autistic disorder (Rutter et al. 2003a). It takes about 90 min to administer this evaluation.

1.4.5   Childhood Autism Rating Scale (CARS)

The Childhood Autism Rating Scale (CARS) was developed by Schopler et al. (1988). This scale is popularly used in India because of its simplicity, conceptual relevance, and high accordance with DSM-IV diagnosis of autism (Russell et al. 2010). This is a 15-item questionnaire that can be used to rate one's behaviour using a 4-point Likert scale ranging from 1 (no signs of autism) to 4 (severe autism). The maximum score is 60. A score ≥ 30.5 and ≤ 37 can be considered to be mild-to-moderate autism. Again, score ≥ 37.5 can be considered to indicate severe autism.

Researchers have proposed that a cut-off of 27 (instead of 30) can be used while administering CARS to adolescents and adults (Mesibov et al. 1989). The CARS is generally used for children aged 2 years and above. This test consists of 14 domains for assessing behaviours associated with autism and a fifteenth domain for rating the general symptoms of autism (Chlebowski et al. 2010). The 14 domains are used to evaluate one in terms of relationship to people, imitation, emotional response, body, use of objects, adaptation to change, visual response, listening response, taste-smell-touch response, fear and nervousness, verbal communication, non-verbal communication, activity level, and consistency in making intellectual response. This scale can be used to differentiate children with autism from those with other developmental delays such as those with intellectual disabilities. This scale can be used to provide scores based on the response from a clinician or teacher or the parent who is acquainted with the child's behaviour.

1.4.6   Checklist for Autism Spectrum Disorders in Toddler (CHAT) and Modified CHAT (M-CHAT)

Among the other deficits, the two deficits that appear early in children at risk of autism are joint attention (Baron-Cohen 1989; Sigman et al. 1986) and pretend play (Wing et al. 1977; Baron-Cohen 1987). Joint attention refers to the ability of a child to establish shared attention towards an object of interest with a social partner using finger pointing, reciprocation through eye gaze, etc. Joint attention skill can be considered as the earliest indicator of a child's mind reading capability in which the child shows sensitivity to what the social partner is interested in or attending to (Baron-Cohen 1991). Pretend play refers to the attribution of imaginary properties to individuals, objects, or events (Leslie 1987). If a child does not demonstrate age-appropriate joint attention and pretend play by the age of 18 months, then the Checklist for Autism Spectrum Disorders in Toddler (CHAT) (Baird et al. 2000) can be used to evaluate whether the child has autism. This checklist consists of two sections having 14 items related to joint attention and pretend play. Out of the 14 items, 9 are in section A of CHAT that is reported by the parents in response to questions asked by the practitioner and 5 are in section B of CHAT that are rated by the practitioner based on direct observation of the child. The purpose of using section B is to validate some of the key responses given by the parent in section A. There are five key items that are related to joint attention and pretend play. Children who fail on all the five key items can be considered to be at greater risk of autism. Additionally, there are some non-key items intended to offer other information so as to distinguish an autistic profile from global developmental delay (Baron-Cohen et al. 2000).

The Modified CHAT (M-CHAT) (Robins et al. 2001) was designed as an autism screening tool for children aged between 16 and 30 months during health check visits (Al-Qabandi et al. 2011). This is a 23-item parent questionnaire with 'yes' or 'no' response options. The M-CHAT actually looks at the expanded form of the parent report questionnaire of the CHAT (Dumont-Mathieu and Fein 2005). This checklist tends to identify children with possible autistic disorder that might also include pervasive developmental disorder—not otherwise specified (PDD-NOS) and not just specifically autistic disorder. Some of the critical items on M-CHAT relate to interest in other children, proto-declarative pointing, bringing in of objects to show those to the parents, imitating, responding to name, and following a pointing gesture.

Both CHAT and M-CHAT are considered to be basic autism screening tools that can be administered to children so as to identify children who are at risk of autism.

1.4.7 Autism Spectrum Screening Questionnaire (ASSQ)

The high-functioning Autism Spectrum Screening Questionnaire (ASSQ) (Ehlers et al. 1999) is a checklist comprising of 27 items used for assessing symptoms that characterize Asperger syndrome and other high-functioning autism spectrum disorders. This is used for children and adolescents with normal intelligence or mild mental retardation. Each item of this Questionnaire uses a 3-point rating scale (0 to 2) with '0' indicating normality, '1' indicating some abnormality and '2' indicating a definite abnormality. The scores can range from 0 to 54. The questionnaire aims to screen one based on social interaction, communication, repetitive behaviour, and clumsiness with regard to motor abilities. This screening tool is generally not used for diagnostic reasons, but can be used to identify children who will need a comprehensive evaluation. Again, ASSQ generally does not work for low-functioning individuals such as those with moderate and severe mental retardation.

In addition, researchers use a revised, extended version of ASSQ (ASSQ-REV) particularly for screening the female phenotype of ASD (Kopp and Gillberg 2011). Added to the 27 items of the ASSQ, the ASSQ-REV has another 18 items that are framed to derive information on the autism phenotype in girls. These include questions on imitation, eating disorders, perception of time, expression of sympathy, determinism, facing difficulties with choosing, particularity on appearance or dress, involvement in activities that might be dangerous, talkative without use of proper facts, etc.

1.5 Summary

This chapter begins by stating the genesis of the term autism. Then, this presents the characteristics that can define autism. Autism-related research is gaining ground given the prevalence of autism. Of course, in certain cases the prevalence rates are dampened due to lack of awareness that can also be attributed to sociocultural issues. However, increased awareness coupled with the availability of appropriate intervention services can be facilitated if one becomes knowledgeable of the autistic symptoms. This is possible if quantitative metrics can be used to assess one's autistic traits. This chapter presents a glimpse of some of the assessment tools proposed by researchers and used by the interventionists.

Once a child's autistic trait has been assessed, the next milestone for the family is to avail the intervention that might address the child's specific need. Conventional intervention techniques have often been proved as powerful. In the next chapter, I will introduce the readers to various aspects of conventional techniques used in different intervention settings.

References

Al-Qabandi M, Gorter JW, Rosenbaum P (2011) Early autism detection: are we ready for routine screening? Paediatrics 128:1–8

APA (2000) Diagnostic and statistical manual of mental disorders: DSM-IV-TR. American Psychiatric Association, Washington, DC

Baird G, Charman T, Baron-Cohen S et al (2000) A screening instrument for autism at 18 months of age: a 6-year follow-up study. J Am Acad Child Adolesc Psychiatry 39(6):694–702

Baron-Cohen S (1987) Autism and symbolic play. Br J Devel Psychol 5:139–148

Baron-Cohen S (1989) Perceptual role-taking and protodeclarative pointing in autism. Br J Devel Psychol 7:113–127

Baron-Cohen S (1991) Precursors to a theory of mind: understanding attention in others. In: Whiten A (ed) Natural theories of mind. Blackwell, Oxford

Baron-Cohen S, Ring HA, Wheelwright S, Bullmore ET, Brammer MJ, Simmons A, Williams SCR (1999) Social intelligence in the normal and autistic brain: an fMRI study. Eur J Neurosci 11 (6):1891–1898

Baron-Cohen S, Sally W, Antony C, Gillian B, Tony C, John S, Auriol D, Peter D (2000) Early identification of autism by the checklist for autism in toddlers (CHAT). J R Soc Med 93:521–525

Bölte S, Poustka F, Constantino JN (2008) Assessing autistic traits: cross-cultural validation of the social responsiveness scale (SRS). Autism Res 1(6):354–363

Bölte S, Westerwald E, Holtmann M, Freitag C, Poustka F (2011) Autistic traits and autism spectrum disorders: the clinical validity of two measures presuming a continuum of social communication skills. J Autism Dev Disord 41:66–72

Cai Y, Chia NK, Thalmann D, Kee NK, Zheng J, Thalmann NM (2013) Design and development of a virtual dolphinarium for children with autism. IEEE Trans Neural Syst Rehabil Eng 21 (2):208–221

Carpenter M, Pennington BF, Rogers SJ (2002) Interrelations among social-cognitive skills in young children with autism. J Autism Dev Disord 32(2):91–106

CDC (2018) Prevalence of autism spectrum disorder among children aged 8 years — autism and developmental disabilities monitoring network, 11 sites, United States, 2014. MMWR Surveill Summ 67(6):1–23

Chlebowski C, Green JA, Barton ML, Fein D (2010) Using the childhood autism rating scale to diagnose autism Spectrum disorders. J Autism Dev Disord 40(7):787–799

Constantino JN (2002) The social responsiveness scale. Western Psych. Serv, California, IL

Constantino JN, Davis SA, Todd RD, Schindler MK, Gross MM, Brophy SL, Metzger LM, Shoushtari CS, Splinter R, Reich W (2003) Validation of a brief quantitative measure of autistic traits: comparison of the social responsiveness scale with the autism diagnostic interview-revised. J Autism Dev Disord 33(4):427–433

Dawson G (2008) Early behavioural intervention, brain plasticity, and the prevention of autism spectrum disorder. Dev Psychopathol 20(3):775–803

Dumont-Mathieu T, Fein D (2005) Screening for autism in young children: the modified checklist for autism in toddlers (M-CHAT) and other measures. Ment Retard Dev Disabil Res Rev 11:253–262

Ehlers S, Gillberg C, Wing L (1999) A screening questionnaire for Asperger syndrome and other high-functioning autism spectrum disorders in school age children. J Autism Dev Disord 29 (2):129–141

Hinnebusch AJ, Miller LE, Fein DA (2017) Autism Spectrum disorders and low mental age: diagnostic stability and developmental outcomes in early childhood. J Autism Dev Disord 47 (12):3967–3982

Jones W, Carr K, Klin A (2008) Absence of preferential looking to the eyes of approaching adults predicts level of social disability in 2-year-old toddlers with autism spectrum disorder. Arch Gen Psychiatry 65(8):946–954

Kanner L (1943) Autistic disturbances of affective contact (PDF). Nervous Child

Kopp S, Gillberg C (2011) The autism spectrum screening questionnaire (ASSQ) – Revised extended version (ASSQ-REV): an instrument for better capturing the autism phenotype in girls? A preliminary study involving 191 clinical cases and community controls. Res Dev Disabil 32:2875–2888

Leslie AM (1987) Pretence and representation: the origins of "theory of mind". Psychol Rev 94:412–426

Lord C, Pickles A, McLennan J, Rutter M, Bregman J, Folstein S, Fombonne E, Leboyer M, Minshew N (1997) Diagnosing autism: analyses of data from the autism diagnostic interview. J Autism Dev Disord 27:501–517

Lord C, Risi S, Lambrecht L, Cook EH, Leventhal BL, DiLavore PC, Pickles A, Rutter M (2000) The autism diagnostic observation schedule-generic: a standard measure of social and communication deficits associated with the spectrum of autism. J Autism Dev Disord 30(3):205–223

McGee GG, Feldman RS, Morrier MJ (1997) Benchmarks of social treatment for children with autism. J Autism Dev Disord 27:353–364

Mesibov GB, Schopler E, Schaffer B, Michal N (1989) Use of the childhood autism rating scale with autistic adolescents and adults. J Am Acad Child Adolesc Psychiatry 28(4):538–541

Moore ST (2002) Asperger syndrome and the elementary school experience: practical solutions for academic and social difficulties. Shawnee Mission, Kansas City, KS

National Statistics Survey (2012) Estimating the prevalence of autism spectrum conditions in adults – Extending the 2007 adult psychiatric morbidity survey, NHS Digital, Official Statistics

Ozonoff S, Goodlin-Jones BL, Solomon M (2005) Evidence-based assessment of autism spectrum disorders in children and adolescents. J Clin Child Adolesc Psychol 34(3):523–540

Robins DL, Fein D, Barton ML et al (2001) The modified checklist for autism in toddlers: an initial study investigating the early detection of autism and pervasive developmental disorders. J Autism Dev Disord 31:131–144

Russell PS, Daniel A, Russell S, Mammen P, Abel JS, Raj LE, Shankar SR, Thomas N (2010) Diagnostic accuracy, reliability and validity of childhood autism rating scale in India. World J Pediatr 6(2):141–147

Rutherford MD, Towns MT (2008) Scan path differences and similarities during emotion perception in those with and without autism spectrum disorders. J Autism Dev Disord 38:1371–1381

Rutter M, Le Couteur A, Lord C (2003a) Autism diagnostic interview revised WPS edition manual. Western Psychological Services, Los Angeles, CA

Rutter M, Bailey A, Berument S, Lord C, Pickles A (2003b) Social communication questionnaire. Western Psychological Services, Los Angeles, CA

Schopler E, Reichier RJ, Renner BR (1988) CARS (the childhood autism rating scale). Western Psychological Services, Los Angeles, CA

Sigman M, Ruskin E (1999) Continuity and change in the social competence of children with autism, down syndrome, and developmental delays. Monogr Soc Res Child Dev 64:11–30

Sigman M, Mundy P, Ungerer J, Sherman T (1986) Social interactions of autistic, mentally retarded, and normal children and their caregivers. J Child Psychol Psychiatry 27:647–656

The Times of India (2012) IIT-G to design learning device for autistic children [Online]. Available http://articles.timesofindia.indiatimes.com/2012-04-05/guwahati/31293580_1_autisticchildren-iit-g-shabina-ahmed

Trepagnier C, Sebrechts MM, Peterson R (2002) Atypical face gaze in autism. CyberPsychol Behav 5(3):213–217

Wing L, Gould J, Yeates SR, Brierley LM (1977) Symbolic play in severely mentally retarded and in autistic children. J Child Psychol Psychiatry 18:167–178

Chapter 2
Conventional Intervention Techniques

2.1 Introduction

Once the autistic traits have been assessed, the next step is to get access to individualized intervention services. There is no denying of the fact that individualized behavioural and educational intervention can be potent to address some of the core social communication deficits characterizing these individuals (NRC 2001). This is because, autism being a spectrum disorder, some of the core deficits can have specific manifestations for each individual. Consequently, each child with autism can be considered to be unique. Thus, this can demand individual-specific intervention to address such disorders. The element of individualization is important for the intervention to be effective.

Again, the expertise and specialized training of the interventionists working with this target group to be able to estimate the affective state of an individual undergoing intervention are critical. This is true, particularly for intervention of individuals with autism who suffer from communication deficits and face difficulties in expressing their affective states. Specifically, these children face milestones in making explicit expression of their affective states. Thus, the success of an intervention aimed to promote skill learning in a child depends on the expertise of the interventionist to infer the affective cues of a child to ensure effective floor-time therapy. The floor-time can be considered as the time in which the caregiver or the therapist can get down to the floor to interact or play with the child at the child's level. This is because the interventionist can use his or her expertise to pick up cues (that are not explicit) from the child so as to get an estimate of the child's affective state. Subsequently, the interventionist can adeptly modify or tune the intervention paradigm so as to suit the

© Springer Nature Switzerland AG 2020
U. Lahiri, *A Computational View of Autism*,
https://doi.org/10.1007/978-3-030-40237-2_2

individual needs of the child. Such specialized intervention can be availed in different settings such as home-based, community-based, and school-based settings.

2.2 Intervention Services in Home-Based Settings

Early intervention can necessarily start in home-based settings. Intervention in home-based settings refers to specialized services delivered either by trained caregivers (e.g. Braiden et al. 2012; Welterlin et al. 2012) or trained interventionists (McConkey et al. 2010) in a home setting. At home-based settings, proper intervention services offered to children with autism by adequately trained caregivers can assist the children to learn skills and also decrease undesirable behaviours in many cases. The home environment can offer an atmosphere to which the child is accustomed, feels safe, and is non-threatened. Offering training in an environment that is familiar to a child might be important since it can help remove elements related to adjusting to a new environment that can be difficult for a child with autism. A home environment can make a child comfortable that can be essential for effective skill learning by the child. Also, the home provides a controlled environment where the caregiver can limit inclusion of distracting elements, thereby helping in uninterrupted learning of behavioural skills. This might be difficult to achieve in settings outside the home environment where the child might need to adjust and share training space with other children. Again, this might become crucial at the initial stages of the intervention and might fade away in the later stages of development. Additionally, a home environment with family members can offer a good setting for training where parents, siblings, and elderly members of the family can participate in the intervention process. This is where joint families having different members of varying age groups become useful. Research has indicated the importance of training the caregivers to carry out intervention in home-based settings particularly at the early stages of a child's development.

There is evidence from the literature that home-based intervention offered by trained caregivers can have positive contributions towards addressing some of the core deficits related to social communication characterizing these children. For example, one of the studies (Perera et al. 2016) reported that the mothers of children (aged 18–40 months) diagnosed with autism were given training by expert clinicians for administering the home-based intervention. This intervention process asked the mother to play with her child for 2 hours per day with each session being 20–30 minutes long. The mother could use symbolic play such as doing simple acts of eating food kept on a plate, drinking soup from a bowl, etc. This can be useful to train the child in various activities of daily living. Specifically, the mother was asked to speak to the child using simple language along with mild physical contact (as appropriate) to draw the child's attention to the specific task. Again, the mother can take the role of task initiator or reciprocate in response to a task done by the child. Since it is known that the child might face difficulty in initiating a task, the mother was asked to initiate the activities in the play at least some of the time.

The idea was to draw the child's attention towards the activities involved in the play and help the child in carrying out symbolic playing. In this way, the caregiver such as the mother can facilitate the child to improve skills in the domains of joint attention (that involves both initiation and reciprocation of joint attention such as through gaze following to triangulate to an object of interest with the social partner), sustained eye contact (this is important since children with autism demonstrate gaze avoidance in which they tend to avoid looking towards the eyes of the social partner), sharing, pointing and requesting, imitating and responding when called by the name, etc. The research findings indicated that promising outcomes were achieved post intervention.

Again, research has shown that home-based Applied Behaviour Analysis (ABA) (details on ABA in Sect. 2.4 below) is often effective for training individuals with autism (Symes et al. 2006) in various activities of daily living. This technique can be used within home-based settings to teach skills related to daily living activities such as feeding oneself, going to bed at a certain time, use bathroom, etc. For example, one of the ways to train a child to maintain a proper bed time can be to ask the child to wear the sleeping suit and take him or her to the bedroom. At the same time, one can create a proper bedtime atmosphere in the child's room by dimming the room lights and turning on a soft music. If this is repeatedly followed for few days, then the child's behaviour with regard to going to bed during the scheduled bedtime will be likely to change and the child will go to bed without being prompted by the mother to do so.

Again, use of social stories in home-based settings can play an important role in the intervention process. The social stories proposed by Carol Gray (1995, 1996) can offer a means to project situations in front of a child with autism in an easy and understandable manner. This in turn can offer information on following context-relevant social protocols. For the sake of individualization, the social stories can be designed to meet individual needs and delivered in an interesting manner in home-based settings while contributing to the skill learning. Social stories can be used to address target behaviour in a home-based setting. The social stories need to be adequately structured. Specifically, this must consist of four types of sentences, namely descriptive, directive, perspective, and control (Gray 1996). Descriptive sentences are those that can describe a social scenario and what can be expected from individuals involved in such a scenario. Directive sentences can be used to help a child to reciprocate with an appropriate response in the social setting. Perspective sentences can be framed to help a child get an idea of the reaction of others in the social situation. Finally, control sentence can be framed to provide relevant clues to help the individual remember the context of the social story. The control sentences can be identified by the individual for whom the story has been developed. Here, I give some examples of social stories along with specific structures that can be used for the social stories.

2.2.1   Example of Teaching the Art of Sharing Through a Social Story

Let us consider a social story being framed to teach a child the art of sharing and the behaviours that can be expected from the child.

The descriptive sentence can refer to a social scenario in which a child is playing with toys within a group (can be siblings of the child) (depicted in Fig. 2.1a). The directive sentence might relate to the child being told that one can expect the child to share the toys with other group members while playing within a group (shown in Fig. 2.1b).

The perspective sentence can be framed to tell the child that when one of the players share a toy with another group member (represented by Fig. 2.1c), then the

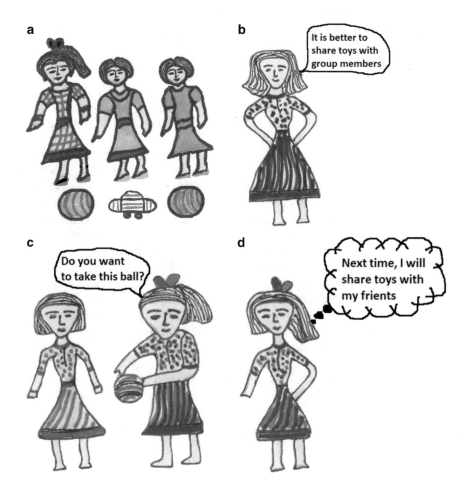

Fig. 2.1 (**a**) Children playing with toys. (**b**) Someone teaching children the art of sharing. (**c**) Sharing a ball with a friend. (**d**) The child thinking that next time she will share toys with her friends

individual will feel happy, smile, and reciprocate by saying 'thank you'. Thus, sharing can be fun. As far as the control sentence is concerned, the child for whom the above story has been framed might say to herself that when she will play with toys (within a group) next time, she will try to share her toys with her partners to have fun (shown by Fig. 2.1d).

2.2.2   Example of Teaching the Art of Initiation of Conversation with Appropriate Reciprocation Through a Social Story

Let us consider a social story designed to teach how one can be expected to initiate a conversation along with appropriate reciprocation in a social setting such as a birthday party. The descriptive sentence can refer to the scenario in which someone is attending a birthday party where various gifts (wrapped in colourful packages) are brought. Also, the gifts are of different sizes, some being large and some small (shown in Fig. 2.2a). The directive sentence can be related to a child being told that when someone goes to a birthday party, then a good way to initiate a conversation with the child (birthday girl) can be to say 'Wish you a very happy birthday. Here is a gift for you' along with handing over the gift to the birthday child (shown in Fig. 2.2b).

The perspective sentence can be to indicate that an appropriate reciprocation by the birthday child would be to say 'thank you' while showing a happy face (represented in Fig. 2.2c). As far as the control sentence is concerned, the child for whom the above story has been framed might say to herself that next time when she will attend a birthday party of her classmate, she will initiate a conversation with the birthday girl and give her a gift. Also, if she invites her friends to her birthday party, then if someone presents her a gift, she will reciprocate by saying 'thank you' with a happy face as a good gesture (shown in Fig. 2.2d).

2.2.3   Example of Teaching Table Manners Through a Social Story

Let us consider a social story that aims to teach table manners while someone is eating food with other members sitting at a table. The descriptive sentence can be designed to present a scenario in which someone is eating breakfast at home while his or her siblings are also sitting at the table (shown in Fig. 2.3a). The directive sentence can be framed to mention to the child that while sitting at a table for having breakfast, it is good manners to say 'hello, good morning to you all', chew food while closing the mouth, make minimal noise with the cutlery while eating and so on (shown in Fig. 2.3b).

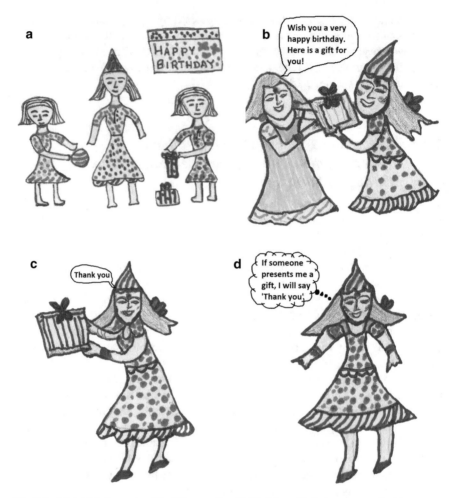

Fig. 2.2 (**a**) A birthday party with different gifts. (**b**) Birthday gifts being presented with conversation initiation. (**c**) Birthday girl reciprocating by saying 'thank you'. (**d**) The child decides that next time she will do similar reciprocation

The perspective sentence can be designed to mention that if someone shows good table manners, then the other members who are also sitting at the table will feel good. On hearing you say 'good morning' they might also say 'good morning to you as well' with a smiling face (shown in Fig. 2.3c). As far as the control sentence is concerned, the child for whom the above story has been framed might utter to herself that next time when she sits with her siblings during breakfast time, she will wish them by saying 'good morning' and sit at the table while following table manners (shown in Fig. 2.3d).

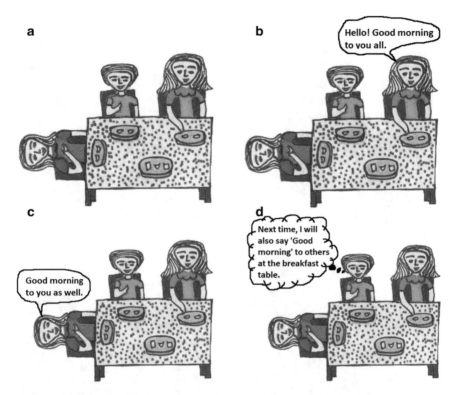

Fig. 2.3 (**a**) Scenario at a breakfast table. (**b**) A member says 'good morning' to others at the table. (**c**) Others reciprocating. (**d**) The child decides that he will follow table manners at the breakfast table

2.2.4   Example of Teaching How to Help Others Through a Social Story

Again, let us consider a social story that is formed to teach the art of helping others and how to communicate while helping others. The descriptive sentence can be formed to present scenarios in which someone might need help or do not need any help. Also, there may be different ways to interact with others to understand if they need any help or not. There can be a scenario in which you can understand that the other person might need help and you can act accordingly. In some cases, it might be difficult to understand whether the other person needs any help from you or not. In such cases, it is better to confirm by asking the person. The directive sentence can be formed to mention to the child that the child need to understand whether the other person needs help, such as for a lady walking with a perambulator and entering the gate of a shopping mall (shown in Fig. 2.4a). In such a case, it would be helpful for the lady if one opens the door for her. In case one is unsure whether the other person (the lady with the perambulator) needs any help, then one can ask 'Do I help you by opening the door for you?' (shown in Fig. 2.4b). The perspective sentence can be

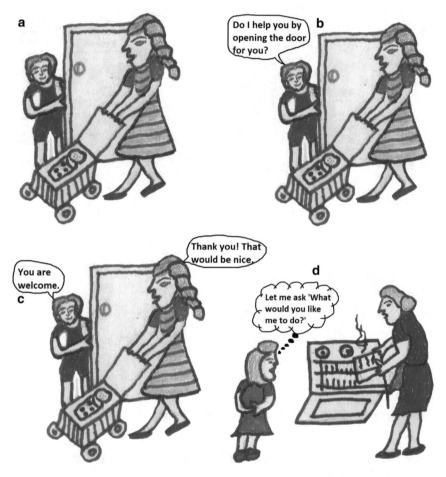

Fig. 2.4 (**a**) A lady with a perambulator entering a shopping mall. (**b**) The boy enquires to find out whether the lady needs help. (**c**) Social communication between the lady and the boy. (**d**) The child thinks that next time she will enquire whether her mother needs any help while using the cooking oven

designed to indicate to the child to try to predict whether someone needs help such as the lady with the perambulator might be thinking that it would be helpful if someone opens the door for her. In such a case if you open the door for her, she will feel good and might say 'Thank you. That would be nice' with a smiling face. In such a case, you can also say 'You are welcome' (Fig. 2.4c).

Again, in case you are unsure whether someone needs help, then to be sure, you can ask the person. If the person says 'No', then that is okay. In case the person says 'Yes', then you might say 'What would you like me to do?' (shown in Fig. 2.4d). As far as the control sentence is concerned, the child for whom the above story has been formed might say to herself that next time if she comes across a situation in which someone needs help, then she would try to help out.

2.2.5   *Example Related to Food Habits Through a Social Story*

Let us consider a social story that is formed to teach how one should eat chewing gum and throw it after use. The descriptive sentence can be designed to present a scenario of someone holding a chewing gum wrapped in a wrapper (shown in Fig. 2.5a). The directive sentence can be formed to mention to the child that it is important that one takes out the chewing gum from the wrapper before putting the chewing gum in the mouth. Also, it is a good habit that one eats the chewing gum while closing the mouth. Again, when the gum has no more flavour, it is better to take it out from the mouth and keep it in the wrapper or tissue paper before throwing it into the dustbin (shown in Fig. 2.5b).

The perspective sentence can be that if you eat the chewing gum with your mouth closed, then you can avoid making a sound and that will be pleasant to others who are sitting close to you. Also, while throwing it off, if you use the wrapper or tissue paper, then the garbage cleaner will not feel bad cleaning the dustbin (represented in Fig. 2.5c). For the control sentence, the child for whom the above story has been formed might say to herself that next time when she will eat chewing gum, she will eat it closing her mouth and would use tissue paper while throwing it off in the dustbin (shown in Fig. 2.5d).

While forming social stories, it has been suggested that one needs to avoid words such as 'I will', 'always', etc. (Gray 1996). Research has shown that the use of social stories can often reduce disruptive behaviour in children with autism (Lorimer et al. 2002).

2.3   Intervention Services in a Community-Based Setting

Intervention at home-based setting facilitates behavioural intervention in a natural environment that is known to the child and most comfortable to the child with autism. However, as they grow, these individuals will need to move out from their comfort zone and interact with the society. For independent living, it is necessary for them to understand the social dynamics that exists in a community. So, it is preferred that the intervention services slowly move outside the home-based setting to community-based setting where the child would need to interact with both known and unknown communicators. Investigators often emphasize the use of such community-based settings for delivering intervention services to the children with autism since this closely resembles the services delivered by practitioners in 'real-world' situations (Williams et al. 2007). The community-based settings can be made structured. The Applied Behaviour Analysis (ABA) therapy offered in such a setting has been shown to be capable of imparting skill learning such as listening skills, social skills, etc. to children with autism. Such settings have also been shown to offer intensive behavioural intervention to individuals with autism (Perrya et al. 2008).

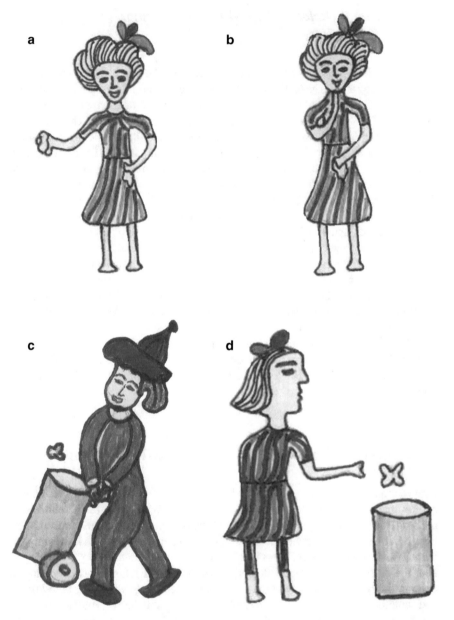

Fig. 2.5 (**a**) A girl holding chewing gum wrapped in a wrapper. (**b**) A girl eating chewing gum while holding the wrapper in her hand. (**c**) Throwing off the chewing gum by putting it in a wrapper so that it is easy for the garbage cleaner. (**d**) The child thinks that she will take precaution while throwing off the chewing gum after eating it

2.3.1   Applied Behaviour Analysis (ABA) Therapy

The Applied Behaviour Analysis (ABA) is often referred to as behaviour therapy (Lovass et al. 1973) or behaviour modification therapy (Martin and Pear 2007). Early intensive behavioural intervention (EIBI) delivered through ABA has been shown to cause improvement in terms of developmental progress and intellectual performance in young children with autism (Lovass 1987; McEachin et al. 1993; Perry et al. 1995; Sallows and Graupner 2005).

Before the therapy is started, a child's skill and level of development is assessed. Thus, specific therapeutic goals are selected in an individualized manner. The therapy regimen can address deficits related to academic, communication, self-care, etc. Then having identified the specific deficit, the task is to break down each into smaller components that can be easily addressed. As the child's development progresses, the skills being taught become more complex.

2.3.1.1   ABA in Educational Programs

In many cases, educational programs rely on the ABA principles to a considerable extent (Foxx 2008). Here, specific skills that need to be taught are identified. This approach facilitates direct teaching of social skills, peer tutoring, program for generalization, etc. The services are delivered in a way that is individualized to a child's specific need.

2.3.1.2   ABA to Prevent Aberrant Behaviour in Children with Autism

The ABA offers scientifically validated methods to overcome obstacles due to a child's aberrant behaviour (Foxx 1982, 1996). In many cases, aberrant behaviour of a child is an acquired one from the child's experience of getting a desired outcome based on the use of the aberrant behaviour. Examples of desired outcome can be drawing attention of others, getting an item that is desired, etc. (Foxx 1996). In many cases, the reasons behind the aberrant behaviour can be environmental, physiological, or social. As a first attempt to treat the aberrant behaviour, the possible reasons need to be identified. For example, a child is displaying aberrant behaviour because he is not feeling well. In that case, proper medication can be given to address the aberrant behaviour.

There are various factors to address aberrant behaviour. The first factor can be developing a hypothesis-driven treatment model (Foxx 1996). Also, the variables that can be used to control the aberrant behaviour need to be identified (Romanczyk 1996). For example, a child might display an aberrant behaviour when he is hungry. Thus, the reason behind his aberrant behaviour needs to be identified. The second factor can be ensuring that a specific stimulus that is leading to the aberrant behaviour is available. For example, one can keep some snacks on hand so that it can be given to the child at times when the aberrant behaviour is likely to occur. The third factor can be a skill-building step. In this, specific favourable behaviour can be taught such as requesting behaviour. For example, in the above case, the child can be taught to request for food whenever he feels hungry. Of course, one needs to be accustomed to the communication style of the child so as to be able to pick up the child's request. The fourth factor can be to avoid occurrence of unpleasant behavioural disposition such as showing frustration, boredom, etc. This can be accomplished by encouraging specific activities such as making a choice. For example, the child can be asked to choose his food item from a food basket. As a fifth factor, the least restrictive treatment modality that is least intrusive but considerably effective can be used. In this, attention is paid to the intensity, severity, rate of occurrence, etc. of aberrant behaviour. As a sixth factor, the aberrant behaviour is not allowed to skip educational activities. Thus, the child is expected to remain in the academic situation before completing the task and finish the activities that he is expected to do. For example, once the child has been given some snacks, he is not allowed to leave the educational activities that he had been doing before completing the tasks allotted to him. For the seventh factor, as the child's behaviour is improving, the complexity of the reinforcement is increased (Foxx 1985a, b). For example, words of appreciation are conveyed to the child in case the child completes the task without demonstrating any aberrant behaviour. As an eighth factor, problem solving is encouraged (Foxx and Bittle 1989). As a ninth factor, the treating professionals are selected and retained for the child since mutual affection is established between the professional and the child. As a tenth factor, the decisions of the child's parents are encouraged since they are the ones who are mostly aware of the child's communication skills, preferences for reinforcers, etc.

2.3.2 Advantages of Community-Based Learning

The community-based learning offers various advantages that are as follows:

2.3.2.1 Structure and Routine

The community-based setting can offer a structured training scenario. The aim of such training is to facilitate the children to follow a specific routine while undergoing intervention in such a setting. Let us consider an example of a classroom environment within a community-based setting. In this, the structure of the setting can be a classroom where toddlers can be taught how to occupy seats in the classroom, use tables for writing, interact with classmates, behave with the teacher, etc. while attending a class. Also, the children can be taught the art of following the class routine such as coming to class in the morning, followed by attending class, understanding that the ringing bell indicates end of class time along with the start of tiffin break, etc.

2.3.2.2   Controllability

The community-based settings can also be used to offer a classroom scenario where the level of distraction in the environment can be controlled. Generally, home-based settings can offer controlled learning environment in which the distractions can be controlled. However, in many real-life situations, when the child is learning a skill, keeping the distraction to a minimum throughout the duration of skill learning might be a challenge. For example, let us consider a home scenario wherein a child with autism named as Hari has few siblings. A teacher has come to teach handwriting to Hari who is sitting in his study room. Also, the mother keeps a watch on the study room of Hari so that his younger siblings do not enter the room and disturb Hari during his study hour. However, due to some preoccupation with a work, the mother of Hari is unable to keep a constant watch and the siblings of Hari come into his room, make noise and go away. This can serve as a distractor to Hari that can deter him from continuing his study. But, if we consider classroom scenarios in schools, achieving full control on any sort of disturbance might be very difficult. So, it is necessary to expose the child to such situations where the disturbance can be systematically manipulated so as to tune Hari to be capable of learning skills while being a part of such situations. This is possible in a community-based setting. If an interventionist at the community-based setting finds that Hari tends to be distracted with noise coming from outside, then, the classroom environment can be modified to offer controlled levels of distraction that can be increased systematically so as to help Hari develop the ability to work even in the presence of distraction. Thus, to start with, the level of distraction is kept less and then in due course, as the child develops coping skills, the level of distraction can be increased. For example, as a first step, the silent classroom environment can be modified to one having light music. Once Hari becomes accustomed to study in such an environment, then the environment can be further modified to systematically increase the level of distraction. One of the ways can be that the members of the community centre walk in and out of that classroom while Hari is studying.

2.3.2.3   Avenue to Interact with Social Partners

It is true that home-based settings offer a known environment to a child where he or she mostly interacts with parents, siblings, etc. all of whom are known to him or her. However, community-based settings can offer a child with an opportunity to interact with both known and unknown communicators. Thus, the child needs to become aware of the social norms and etiquettes while communicating with individuals who are unknown to him or her. Also, the child attending the community-based centre gets an opportunity to have a first-hand knowledge of the sense of social relationships.

2.3.2.4 Provides variety of Experiences

A community-based setting can offer one with the opportunity to get a variety of experiences while interacting with different members of the community. While being a part of a community centre, the child will be expected to interact with different individuals possessing different attributes. Thus, this can offer an avenue of generalization. This is particularly important for children with autism who possess cognitive challenges and thereby face difficulty in generalizing experience or the art of transferring knowledge across various situations.

2.4 Intervention Services in School-Based Settings

Individuals with ASD are often characterized by atypical behaviour. Interventions offered in school-based settings often use combinations of behavioural or developmental techniques. The Applied Behaviour Analysis (ABA) (Lindgren and Doobay 2012) is one of these techniques. The ABA techniques use a closed-loop approach that seeks to apply behavioural principles with an aim to (1) change specific behaviours and (2) evaluate the effectiveness of the intervention. This is necessary because autism is a spectrum disorder. Thus, a technique that might work for one child may not be suitable for another child. This technique pays attention to both the social and physical environments in which the child resides. The specialized intervention services are generally offered by a trained behavioural psychologist or behaviour analyst. Given the spectrum nature of the disorder, different instructional procedures (e.g. prompt delivery, shaping, fading) are offered within ABA depending on the context and the unique characteristics of the child receiving the intervention (Harrower and Dunlap 2001). Different approaches, such as intense, structured approaches (e.g. discrete trial training), naturalistic approaches (e.g. functional communication training, pivotal response training), and self-management procedures (Iovannone et al. 2003) are used while delivering this intervention.

2.4.1 Instructional Procedures Used Within ABA

2.4.1.1 Prompt Delivery

Individuals with autism often need external stimulus, such as a prompt to begin or to terminate a particular behaviour. Here, we discuss the use of appropriate verbal, physical or visual cues or prompts with an aim to encourage a child to demonstrate a desirable behaviour. For example, if a child, Shyam (say) is to be told to place his book on a shelf, then the teacher can use a verbal prompt by saying 'Hello Shyam. Can you please keep the book on the shelf?' Instead, the teacher can use physical

Fig. 2.6 A teacher using
prompting gesture as a
prompt towards a book shelf

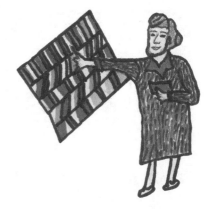

Fig. 2.7 A picture card
showing a smiling face

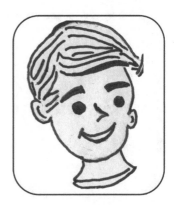

prompt by using a pointing gesture towards the shelf indicating the child Shyam to
place the book on the shelf (Fig. 2.6).

If required, the teacher can use a combination of verbal and physical prompts. In
recent times, the therapists also suggest use of auditory prompting to offer auditory
cue for in-class self-monitoring to diminish off-task behaviour in a classroom (Coyle
and Cole 2004).

In certain cases, the teacher can use a visual prompt such as while teaching
emotion recognition skill to children with autism. Being able to express emotion is
valuable for carrying on social communication. However, children with autism face
milestones while showing and recognizing emotional expressions. Also, it is well
known that children with autism are mostly good visual learners. Thus, often
teachers use visual prompts for these children. Let us consider a situation in which
the teacher is trying to teach the child Shyam how to show a smiling face. In this
case, the teacher can use a visual prompt by showing a picture card having a smiling
face drawn on it (Fig. 2.7 shows such an example).

Sometimes a number of picture cards can be used to teach activities of daily living
to a child with autism in which the child needs to carry out a sequence of activities.
For example, a teacher can teach the sequence of activities involved in brushing of

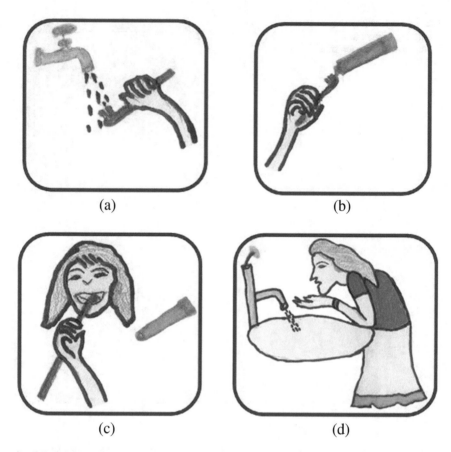

Fig. 2.8 Picture cards to teach the brushing of teeth

teeth. Thus, the teacher can use the audio-visual mode of prompt delivery. In this, the teacher can use a sequence of picture cards while arranging these in order and narrating each task. The first step can be to open the tap and rinse the brush followed by closing the tap (Fig. 2.8a). The next task can be to open the toothpaste tube and add the paste on the bristles of the brush (Fig. 2.8b). The third step can be to close the toothpaste tube and brush the teeth (Fig. 2.8c). The fourth step can be to open the tap and wash the brush followed by washing the mouth with water and closing the tap (Fig. 2.8d).

2.4.1.2 Shaping

This technique aims to change one's behaviour gradually and systematically by offering scaffolded reinforcement. For example, if the target behaviour is to encourage a child named as Bipin (say) to sit in a group (of children) during lunch hour, then such a target behaviour can be shaped gradually and sequentially (expressed as steps here). Thus, during the lunch hour, if Bipin is standing close to a group, then such a behaviour exhibited by Bipin can be appreciated by praising Bipin (first step). Such praise can serve as a reinforcer. In case Bipin is found to stand inside the group, then as a next step, Bipin's improved behaviour can be applauded (serving as a reinforcer). Finally, if Bipin sits inside the group and enjoys the lunch with his friends, then the final reinforcer can be used.

Again, prompting through stimulus shaping is another approach. This has been shown to be powerful in teaching visuo-motor skills (Mosk and Bucher 1984). In this study, two tasks were used, namely the peg-board task and a self-care task. The peg-board task required one to place two pegs at two holes of a peg board. First, only a verbal instruction was delivered. If the child was not able to correctly respond to the instruction, then the prompt was shaped until the child was successful in completing the task. The shaped prompts can be verbal instruction with pointing, followed by verbal instruction with physical prompt, followed by verbal instruction with hand-over-hand prompting, etc. The physical prompt can be delivered through lightly touching the hand of the child. The hand-over-hand prompt in the case of peg-board task can be holding the hand of the child to pick up the peg and insert it in the hole of the peg-board.

2.4.1.3   Fading

This technique refers to gradual decrease in the extent of prompting needed to facilitate a child to complete a task. The idea is that the facilitator needs to systematically reduce the assistance in helping a child while doing a task. The ultimate aim is to make the child independent while executing the task (Alberto and Troutman 2006). For example, let us consider that a child with autism named as Thomas (say) needs to be taught to have his tiffin during the scheduled tiffin break at the school. As a first step, when the bell rings to announce the tiffin break, the teacher displays a photo of a child opening his tiffin box and eating his tiffin. This will be added by a verbal prompt with the teacher saying 'Hello Thomas, this is tiffin break. Please open your tiffin box and have your tiffin' (Fig. 2.9a). If Thomas can follow the teacher's prompt, then the teacher can offer a reinforcer such as verbal praise. After a few days, when the teacher plans to fade her prompt, once the bell rings for the tiffin break, she only displays the photo, but does not add any verbal prompt (Fig. 2.9b). If Thomas takes out his tiffin box and starts eating even with the faded prompt, the teacher can add a reinforcer. Lastly, once the teacher finds that Thomas is able to understand the tiffin break, she further fades her prompt by walking out of the classroom when the tiffin bell rings and looks at whether Thomas is eating his tiffin. As a reinforcer, she can hand him a small gift (Fig. 2.9c).

Again, fading prompt in terms of script-fading is common and is important for teaching communication skills to children with autism (Sarokoff and Taylor 2001). In this study, verbal instructions followed by packages with embedded text were offered to individuals with autism. One could eat food item or play video game kept

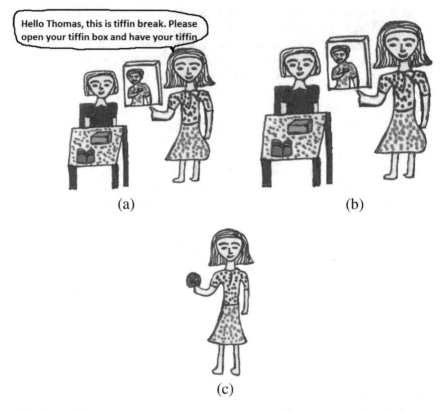

Fig. 2.9 Using fading prompt

in packages. In this, a five-step script-fading prompt (Krantz and McClannahan 1993) without verbal prompting was used. The children were asked to sit across each other and read the text aloud. In Step 1, 25% of the words were faded out from back to front. In Step 2, half of each sentence was faded out. In Step 3, the package (of the item) and the first letter of each line of text remained. In Step 4, the paper was presented with the package. In Step 5, only the package remained. Results indicated that post few exposures, in spite of the faded text, the children could communicate with each other and this continued even under novel conditions.

2.4.2   Approaches Used within ABA

2.4.2.1   Discrete Trial Training (DTT)

This is based on behavioural learning theory and Applied Behaviour Analysis (ABA). This aims to train a child to demonstrate appropriate behaviours in the context of learning language, motor skills, imitation and play, expressing emotions, etc. The Discrete Trial Training (DTT) can be used for teaching new discriminations (such as giving the correct response to requests made), speech sounds, and motor-related skills. Also, this can be used to teach one advanced skills and to manage disruptive behaviour.

2.4.2.1.1 New Discriminations

In this, a facilitator presents a discriminative stimulus to the child. If the child reciprocates with an appropriate response to the cue given by the teacher, then the facilitator encourages the child by using a reward (as a consequence). For example, if a teacher holds up a ball and asks 'What is this?', the correct response in this case is 'ball' and not 'car'. In the same way, if the teacher holds up a car and asks the child 'What is this?', the correct response from the child needs to be 'car' and not 'ball'. When implementing the DTT, the teacher can use cueing, prompting, fading, etc. as appropriate for the child. Thus, when the ball is shown to the child, the correct response is 'ball'. If the child has mastered the correct response of saying the word 'ball', then the teacher uses the same process to teach the second word 'car'. Once the child has mastered the second response, the teacher alternates the cues while alternately holding up the ball and the car and asking the child to respond. This is to ensure whether the child has learnt to discriminate between the two items, such as ball and car (in this case). This approach can be used to teach various skills.

2.4.2.1.2 Imitation

This refers to a response that is identical to the given cue. An example can be clapping when the teacher is also clapping. Training in imitation skills is important for children with autism because they are often characterized by difficulties in imitating others. By this approach, a child can be taught to do different tasks while seeing and imitating the teacher.

2.4.2.1.3 Receptive Language

This refers to executing an action in response to a verbal cue delivered by the teacher. For example, let us consider a scenario in which various play items such as ball, toy car, etc. are lying on the floor. Now if the teacher says the ball, the child is expected to pick up the ball. In case, the teacher says the car, the child is expected to pick up the car. Such training is important for children with autism because they mostly lack the receptive language or demonstrate delays in the development of this skill.

2.4.2.1.4   Conversation

This refers to giving verbal responses to verbal cues. Specifically, this expects a child to respond to a statement with another statement on the same topic asked. For example, let us consider a scenario in which a blue-coloured ball is lying on a table and the teacher asks 'What is this?' The child responds by saying 'This is a blue-coloured ball'.

2.4.2.1.5   Sentence, Grammar, and Syntax

This refers to use of language to describe relationships between objects. The DTT is mostly used in extending the ability of a child from uttering words to speaking sentences (Risley et al. 1972). For example, let us consider a scenario in which two balls, one red-coloured small ball and a blue-coloured larger ball, are lying on the floor. If the teacher points towards these balls and asks a child 'What are these?', the child is expected to learn to respond by saying that 'This is a red-coloured ball and this is smaller than the blue-coloured ball'.

2.4.2.1.6   Alternative Communication Systems

In certain cases, children face difficulties in making use of spoken language irrespective of the instructional approach. In such cases, the teacher can encourage the child to use alternative communication modes such as use of sign language, picture communication systems, etc. In the picture communication system, the child might be encouraged to use picture cards to communicate what they want. For example, let us consider a scenario in which the child is thirsty and she wants to have a glass of water. Then, the child will choose a picture card showing a glass of water and hand it over to the teacher to indicate that she is thirsty and wants the teacher to hand over a glass of water to her.

2.4.2.1.7   Management of Disruptive Behaviour

Research has investigated ways of managing disruptive behaviours as commonly exhibited by children with autism by replacing such behaviour with alternate or adaptive behaviour (Matson et al. 1996). For example, let us consider a situation in which a child always throws tantrums if she wants a particular object. This is a disruptive behaviour and the teacher might teach her an alternative behaviour such as asking the child to verbally request for the object (instead of throwing tantrums).

2.4.2.2   Functional Communication Training (FCT)

Several researchers (Carr and Durand 1985; Durand and Merges 2001; Wacker et al. 1990) have used Functional Communication Training (FCT) to address communication and behavioural needs of children with autism. This involves identification of the function of a behaviour followed by replacing the challenging behaviour with an appropriate communicative response that serves to do the same function. In this, the first step is conducting interviews, making direct observation and functional analysis by the teacher so as to come up with a hypothesis explaining the function associated with the behaviour. The next step is to find out an appropriate communicative response based on whether a child is non-verbal or verbal. After the type of response has been selected, the next step is to teach the communicative response to the child (Lalli et al. 1995).

If a child named as Ann (say) with autism is non-verbal, then the interventionist can take the help of picture cards to communicate with Ann. Let us consider a scenario where a teacher wants to teach Ann the steps involved in brushing her teeth after getting out of bed. The teacher verbally says the steps while displaying picture cards showing photos such as a child holding a brush in one hand and the toothpaste tube in the other hand, a child brushing her teeth, washing her mouth by using the tap water from a basin. All of these picture cards are preferably coupled with verbal messages. Now to ensure that Ann has understood the steps, the teacher can say that 'I have finished brushing my teeth. What should I do next?' Simultaneously, the teacher will display all the picture cards showing the steps involved in brushing the teeth in front of Ann. If Ann points towards the picture card displaying a person washing her mouth by using the tap water from a basin, then, the teacher can say that 'You are correct. Now I need to wash my mouth by using the tap water from a basin'.

Again, let us consider a scenario in which Ann is verbal and the teacher wants to encourage Ann to use a verbal mode of communication. Say, the teacher finds that Ann is standing alone outside the classroom. Also, the teacher knows that Ann likes toy cars. Now, the teacher walks over to Ann and shows her three picture cards, one showing a photo of a car and the other two showing photos of the scooter and cycle. Then the teacher asks Ann 'Which one among these three would you like to have?' If Ann points towards the picture card showing the photo of a car, then the teacher says 'OK'. However, if instead of pointing towards the picture card, Ann says 'Car', then the teacher says 'Great! Here is your toy car' and hands over a toy car to Ann as a reward.

The final step in FCT can be ignoring the challenging behaviour and acknowledging or appreciating the desired communicative behaviour that can replace the challenging behaviour. For example, a child is throwing tantrums to get a particular object. In such a case, the teacher might ignore the challenging behaviours that is the tantrum. Instead, the teacher might prompt the child to take a break. After the break, when the child displays the correct communicative response, the teacher acknowledges this behaviour and hands over the object that the child wanted.

2.4.2.3 Pivotal Response Training (PRT)

The Pivotal Response Training (PRT) involves systematic strategies to address deficits in target behaviours. The idea is to enhance one's pivotal learning in terms of motivation to do a task while using proper communication, responding to multiple but simultaneous cues, initiating conversation, managing oneself in daily living tasks, and also learning to empathize. Generally, a natural setting is recommended for administering this training. One often sees a reduction in behavioural disturbances post training.

The PRT can be implemented in different settings such as special inclusion schools by peers, home-based settings by parents, etc. In this, different scoring mechanisms are employed to score the behaviour of a child undergoing the PRT (Pierce and Schreibman 1995). For example, focus is given on whether the child being trained is maintaining interaction, initiating interaction or initiating play.

2.4.2.3.1 Maintaining Interaction

This checks whether the child with autism is capable of maintaining the same verbal or non-verbal activity as the peer. If the child can comply with the request made by the peer, then the child is scored as maintaining the interaction. In contrast, if the child does not allow the peer to take his turn, then the child is scored as not maintaining interaction. For example, let us consider a child is playing with a ball along with his peer. In this process, if the child does not throw the ball towards his peer but continuously keeps the ball in his possession, then the child is not considered to maintain interaction.

2.4.2.3.2 Initiating Interaction

Any verbalization that may not be considered as a response to the previous question can be thought of as initiating interaction. For example, if the child says 'I like ice cream', then this is considered as initiating interaction.

2.4.2.3.3 Initiating Play

This refers to the initiation of a verbal or non-verbal request for a new game or play item. For example, if a child is engaged in playing with a ball and says 'play ball' to his peer or hands over a ball to his peer, then the child is scored as 'initiating play'.

Again, let us consider an example in which a therapist is participating with a child in a block puzzle game while administering PRT. To start communication, sometimes the therapist places a block in the hands of the child. Again, to encourage the child to initiate a conversation, sometimes the therapist hides a block of the puzzle under a carpet and waits for the child to ask her for the block. Say, the child is making a house out of the blocks and the therapist finds that the door to the house is missing, then the therapist starts giving verbal cues to the child by saying that 'where is the door to enter the house?' The therapist waits for the child to continue playing the block puzzle while building the house with its windows, chimneys, etc. using his imagination. In this way, the child goes on to build a house, a small dog, a courtyard, etc. with the help of the blocks. As the play time increases, the therapist can understand that the child has become tired, but is still continuing with the block puzzle game as he is interested in playing with it. In such a case, the therapist can point towards the dog built by the child and tell that the dog (with personification) is tired and it is bedtime for his pet dog. The idea is to help the child to understand that the game should be stopped since it is his bedtime.

2.4.2.4   Social Skills Training (SST)

Children with ASD are often characterized by deficits in social interaction. The SST is a way to address this deficit in the children with ASD. The idea is to train a child in healthy social skills so that his or her prosocial behaviour can increase. One of the important tools that can facilitate in nurturing social skills in these children is using social narrative or story. The SST can be peer-mediated and/or therapist-mediated. For encouraging peer-mediated intervention, one can offer a school environment to the child where the child gets to meet his or her peers who can serve as important agents in social play. The therapist-mediated SST consists of one-on-one intervention sessions in which the therapist can offer focused training to the child while addressing different aspects of social interaction skills. For example, the therapist can address aspects such as eye contact, joint attention, initiation of communication, etc.

2.4.2.5   Cognitive Behavioural Therapy (CBT)

The Cognitive Behavioural Therapy (CBT) aims to replace negative thoughts and behaviours of a child with improved mood, to facilitate the child to acquire adaptive functioning skills. This therapy is important for children with autism since anxiety disorders are often seen in these children, and this is often coupled with impairment in social functioning (Bellini 2004; De Bruin et al. 2007). The impairment in social and school (or occupational) functioning can be a prevalent consequence of such a disorder.

A crucial part of this therapy is thought tracking by the therapist. The therapist and a child identify maladaptive cognition through discussion and questioning. For example, the child might say that 'I cannot do the task by myself, since if I do the task on my own, my friends will never help me'. This is followed by questioning the maladaptive cognition. Thus, the therapist can ask the question 'Would they really not help you with anything else?' This can be followed by restructuring the cognitive behaviour by uttering to oneself by saying 'Even if I do the task by myself, my friends will probably help me with the tasks that I still need help'. Thus, this can be used to improve a child's daily living skills. The caregivers can also be trained to help their child gain independence through communication such as by offering choices, providing positive feedback, and offering reinforcement for a task that has been well accomplished.

If a child is disturbed due to some reason, the therapist questions the child while digging deeper to find the basis of the thought that has been disturbing the child. Let us consider an example. Let us consider that a child named as Sonu (say) is sitting on a chair at one corner of a playground where other children of similar age are playing. The therapist tries to dig deep by questioning to find out the reason behind his staying aloof from the other children. Thus, a therapist performing CBT might ask him 'Why are you not playing with your friends and sitting on this chair alone?' To this, Sonu might say that 'I do not like to play with others'. Then the therapist might ask 'What is the reason that you do not like to play with your friends?' Sonu might say that 'Somehow I feel left out of the group since these children might speak bad about me if I go to play with them'. Then the therapist digs deeper by asking Sonu that 'Why will they say bad about you?' To this, Sonu might respond by saying that 'At times I behave unnaturally and that is not in my control'. In turn, the therapist might ask 'Why do you behave unnaturally? Can you realize that the way you behave is unnatural?' In this way, the therapist goes deeper to find out the very basis of the thought disturbing Sonu that is preventing him to play with other children. Then the therapist can suggest different strategies to handle such progression in disturbing thoughts. One of the strategies can be to speak to oneself 'STOP this thought'. This therapy is often used for individuals with autism.

2.5 Conventional Intervention Services: Advantages and Some Milestones in an Indian Setting

Conventional intervention services have been shown to be potent in offering skill training to children with autism. The intensive training can thus bring changes in the functional abilities of a child with autism and in turn are a boon to families having such children.

Here, I discuss some of the advantages and limitations of conventional intervention services.

2.5.1 Advantages of Conventional Intervention Services

Some of the biggest advantages of conventional intervention techniques are as follows:

2.5.1.1 Individualization

Given the spectrum nature of the disorder, individualization of intervention service is critical for it to be effective. By individualized services, I mean that one must understand the specific requirements of a child and choose an intervention that is appropriate for the specific child. Each child with autism being unique, appropriate use of specific intervention approaches to cater to the child's individualized vulnerabilities is very important. The individualized services that might be effective for a child need to be decided based on comprehensive assessment. What works well for one child may not be appropriate for another child.

Also, the type and specifics of the intervention might be adapted to the time-sensitive requirements of the child. For example, as training of a child progresses, an intervention strategy that worked for the child when he or she was young may need to be modified as he or she grows older. In other words, the intervention paradigm has to be tuned to suit the child's specific intervention needs for effective floor-time therapy. For example, for a toddler having sleep issues, the therapist can adopt ways to convey that it is bedtime at the end of a game-play session by showing a toy doll as trying to lie down for going to sleep. However, when the specific toddler grows a bit older, the therapist might want to address his issues associated with activities of daily living such as getting ready for school in the morning. For imparting such daily living skills, the therapist might use a visual schedule to teach the child that he needs to brush his teeth, take a shower, put on the school dress, have breakfast, and get ready for school.

Thus, for a targeted intervention to be effective for a specific child, it is very important that there must be a regular collection of data and noting down of the observations on the child's progress. This needs to be coupled with the continuous assessment of the response to intervention to ensure whether the intervention services designed for the specific child are effective.

2.5.1.2 Physical Embodiment

In conventional intervention, the specialized services are offered by the human therapists. Such intervention often involves several hours of one-on-one sessions with the trained therapists at the institution, home, etc. Thus, the therapist's presence can offer a 3D-embodied presence of an external agent in the child's living space. In other words, the embodied presence can bring in connectivity with real-life situations in which a child needs to communicate with social communicators. Thus, the physical presence of the therapist in the training environment of a child can offer the senses of human contact, interaction, and relationship that can be important for comprehensive social communication skill learning, particularly relevant for children with autism.

2.5.1.3 Variations in the Child's Daily Life

Healthy community living needs one to make friendship, build relations, share thoughts, etc. with others. However, children with autism often like to be in their own little world while being alienated from the society. The child might use his or her own mode of communication to communicate with his or her parents and siblings who might have already practised the art of deciphering the mode used by the child to communicate. But to an outsider, decoding the intended message of the child might be difficult. The physical presence of a therapist in the child's world during the therapy sessions can bring in variations in the child's world by exposing the child to individuals whom the child does not know (at least during the initial training sessions).

2.5.2 Limitations of Conventional Intervention Services in the Indian context

Though promising, each of the conventional techniques faces certain milestones, particularly in countries with developing economy such as India. Some of these milestones are:

2.5.2.1 Cost of Intervention

It has been well accepted that early intensive intervention is beneficial for children with autism. Often, the children go through a number of therapies such as speech therapy, behaviour therapy, arts-based therapy, yoga therapy, etc. Mostly the intervention requires long hours of therapy sessions that need dedicated presence of a therapist. Thus, the therapy sessions often become quite costly. The situation in India is also grim. Depending on the type of intervention services, the costs can be Rs. 30,000 to Rs. 40,000 per month. These costs refer to the direct costs incurred in providing therapy for the child.

Added to this, there is latent cost that can be referred to as the indirect cost. For example, often it is seen that the mother of a child with autism accompanies the child while taking him or her to the therapy centre and spends time with her child. In such cases, since most of her time goes into supporting the child, the mother cannot earn her own living. This can get reflected as an indirect cost.

In short, the high cost of intervention often makes specialized intervention inaccessible for the majority of households having such children.

2.5.2.2   Observation-Based Techniques

Each child with autism is unique. This necessitates the use of individualized intervention services. Often, expert therapists use observation-based techniques to get an estimate of the child's affective state such as whether the child is anxious or is not paying attention during the skill learning session. In turn, the therapist can change the intervention paradigm so as to bring back the child's engagement with the task at hand.

In other words, the trained therapist needs to be adept in picking up cues demonstrated by the child using observation-based techniques. Then the therapist can ensure floor-time therapy that is important for effective skill learning (Wieder and Greenspan 2005). Often the observation-based techniques are not quantitative in nature and can be subjective. Thus, the quality of assessment of the autistic traits can also depend to a large extent on a therapist's expertise to pick up the subtle cues from the child.

2.5.2.3   Resource Limitation

Since the conventional intervention services are mostly exclusively dependent on human therapists who are specially trained in these services, scarcity in the availability of such trained manpower might adversely affect the delivery of such services. This is the scenario in many parts of the world including India. With increasing awareness towards autism and the need for early intervention, parents of such children try their best to avail such services for their child.

However, the delivery of autism intervention services is often restricted by the availability of special needs schools and intervention centres. This is particularly true in developing countries like India, where the autism intervention centres are mostly localized within selected pockets of the urban community. In many cases, parents have to commute large distances for availing specialized intervention services. Often the special needs schools are limited and some of those which are available are mostly run by consortiums formed by parents of these children. Additionally, there is a reduced availability of adequately trained therapists. Such resource limitations often adversely affect the families of these children who often face difficulties in providing specialized intervention services to their child.

2.5.2.4   Paucity in Training Materials

Children with autism undergoing therapy are often exposed to various training modules that focus on different aspects of daily living skills. For this, different training materials are required. Sometimes, the training materials can be in the form of coloured balls, multi-coloured beads, pictures drawn on cards, symbols drawn on paper, etc. Often, the therapists put in hard work to create such training materials that might need to be individualized based on a child's specific need. Again, the children undergoing intervention can have varying levels of functional capability. Specifically, some of them can be low functioning and some can be high functioning with varying speech capabilities. Children with limited speech often use alternate modes of communication such as picture cards displaying symbols or photos.

For example, if a child with limited speech capability is feeling thirsty, then, the child might show a picture card displaying the image of a glass of water to the teacher who in turn can interpret that the child is thirsty and hand him or her a glass of water. Also, in many cases, the picture cards can be used by a teacher to offer training to a child. For example, if a therapist is trying to teach the art of recognizing emotion, such as 'happy', then the therapist can show a picture card displaying a smiling face of a girl and tell that 'This is a smiling face. It looks like she is happy'. In many cases, the use of visuals such as picture cards becomes important, since it is well known that children with autism are often visual learners. These training materials are often manually prepared and in many cases these might be of limited variety.

2.5.2.5 Limited Variations in Training Situations

Children with autism are often characterized by deficits in their ability to generalize. In other words, once certain skills are taught to them within a particular context, they find it difficult to transfer the skills learnt to another scenario. For example, if a child is taught the tips on having proper social communication in a school-based controlled setting and then they are exposed to a social gathering such as a playground or a park environment, they might find it difficult to carry out social communication with their peers in such a scenario. In such a case, it might be useful to expose the children to such real-life situations while imparting social communication skills to the child. At the same time, one needs to ensure safety while exposing the child to such real-life settings.

For example, if a child needs to be taught the way in which he or she is expected to interact with peers in a park environment, it might be useful for the child to be taught the art of communication while being in such an environment. However, exposing the child to such an environment during the training session might not be safe for the child because the child might not be able to transfer the tips on social communication taught to him at school to the real-life park environment. This might result in the child making inappropriate reciprocation causing the child not to be accepted by his or her peers. At the same time, giving a realistic experience while immersing the child in the real-life social scenario can be important.

One of the ways to achieving this while ensuring safety of the child in the training process is to simulate such real-life scenarios within controlled settings and give the child immersion into such scenarios. It might not be feasible to simulate various social situations at the therapist's clinic due to resource limitations. Also, offering variations in controlled settings might be challenging in many cases that in turn restricts variation in the design of training scenarios.

2.6 Summary

In this chapter, I have introduced the reader to the different approaches used by the conventional intervention used in home-based, community-based, and school-based settings. Also, the importance of conventional approaches in adhering to the individualization of the intervention services to ensure effective floor-time therapy was emphasized. Though powerful, the conventional techniques suffer from certain limitations such as restricted availability of adequately trained therapists, limited specialized intervention units, high cost of one-on-one intervention services, limited variations in the training scenarios, etc.

Thus, the next question that is coming to my mind is, so what next? Can there be alternative modalities? Since the conventional intervention approaches are powerful, how about taking the knowledge learnt from the conventional approaches and instilling that to alternate approaches that can offer complementary solutions? With technological progress, the thought that is coming to me is how about using technology? Yes, it is necessary to understand the scope of alternate technology-assisted intervention approaches that can serve as complementary tools in the hands of the therapists. In the next chapter, I will try to introduce the reader to some of the technology-assisted intervention platforms that are slowly gaining ground while considering the global scenario.

References

Alberto PA, Troutman AC (2006) Applied behavior analysis for teachers, 7th edn. Pearson Education, Upper Saddle River, NJ

Bellini S (2004) Social skill deficits and anxiety in high-functioning adolescents with autism spectrum disorder. Focus Autism Other Dev Disabil 19:78–86

Braiden HJ, McDaniel B, McCrudden E, Hanes M, Crozier B (2012) A practice-based evaluation of Barnardo's forward steps early intervention programme for children diagnosed with autism. Child Care Pract 18:227–242

Carr EG, Durand VM (1985) Reducing behavior problems through functional communicationtraining. J Appl Behav Anal 18:111–126

Coyle C, Cole P (2004) A videotaped self-modeling and self-monitoring treatment program to decrease off-task behavior in children with autism. J Intellect Develop Disabil 29:3–15

De Bruin EI, Ferdinand RF, Meester S, de Nijs PF, Verheij F (2007) High rates of psychiatric co-morbidity in PDD-NOS. J Autism Dev Disord 37(5):877–886

Durand VM, Merges E (2001) Functional communication training: a contemporary behavior analytic intervention for problem behaviors. Focus Autism Other Dev Disabil 16:110–119

Foxx RM (1982) Decreasing the behaviours of persons with severe retardation and autism. Research Press, Champaign, IL

Foxx RM (1985a) The Jack Tizzard memorial lecture: decreasing behaviors: clinical, ethical, legal, and environmental issues. Aust N Z J Dev Disabil 10:189–199

Foxx RM (1985b) Social skills training: the current status of the field. Aust N Z J Dev Disabil 10:237–243

Foxx RM (1996) Twenty years of applied behaviour analysis in treating the mosrt severe problem behaviour: lessons learned. Behav Anal 19(2):225–235

Foxx RM (2008) Applied behavior analysis treatment of autism: the state of the art. Child Adolesc Psychiatr Clin N Am 17:821–834

Foxx RM, Bittle RG (1989) Thinking it through: teaching a problem solving strategy for community living. Research Press, Champaign, IL

Gray CA (1995) Teaching children with autism to "read" social situations. In: Quill KA (ed) Teaching children with autism: strategies to enhance communication and socialization. Delmar, Albany, NY, pp 219–241

Gray CA (1996) Social stories and comic strip conversations: Unique methods to improve social understanding [Videotape]. Future Horizons, Arlington, TX

Harrower JK, Dunlap G (2001) Including children with autism in general education classrooms: a review of effective strategies. Behav Modif 25:762–784

Iovannone R, Dunlap G, Huber H, Kincaid D (2003) Effective educational practices for students with autism spectrum disorders. Focus Autism Other Dev Disabil 18:150–165

Krantz PJ, McClannahan LE (1993) Teaching children with autism to initiate to peers: effects of a script-fading procedure. J Appl Behav Anal 26:121–132

Lalli JS, Casey S, Kates K (1995) Reducing escape behavior and increasing task completion with functional communication training, extinction, and response chaining. J Appl Behav Anal 28:261–268

Lindgren SD, Doobay DA (2012) Evidence-based interventions for autism spectrum disorders. Curr Probl Pediatr Adolesc Health Care 48(10):234–249

Lorimer PA, Simpson RL, Myles BS, Ganz JB (2002) The use of social stories as a preventative behavioral intervention in a home setting with a child with autism. J Posit Behav Interv 4 (1):53–60. First Published January 1, 2002

Lovass OI (1987) Behavioural treatment and normal educational and intellectual functioning in young autistic children. J Consult Clin Psychol 55:3–9

Lovass OI, Koegel RL, Simmons JQ et al (1973) Some generalization and follow-up measures on autistic children in behaviour therapy. J Appl Behav Anal 6:131–165

Martin G, Pear JB (2007) Behavior modification: what it is and how to do it, 8th edn. Prentice Hall, Upper Saddle River, NJ

Matson J, Benavidez D, Compton L, Paclawskyj T, Baglio C (1996) Behavioral treatment of autistic persons: a review of research from 1980 to the present. Res Dev Disabil 17:433–465

McConkey R, Truesdale-Kennedy M, Crawford H, McGreevy E, Reavey M, Cassidy A (2010) Preschoolers with autism spectrum disorders: evaluating the impact of a home-based intervention to promote their communication. Early Child Dev Care 180:299–315. https://doi.org/10.1080/03004430801899187

McEachin JJ, Smith TH, Lovass OI (1993) Long-term outcome for children with autism who received early intensive behavioural treatment. Am J Ment Retard 97(40):359–372

Mosk MD, Bucher B (1984) Prompting and stimulus shaping procedures for teaching visual-motor skills to retarded children. J Appl Behav Anal 17:23–34

NRC (2001) Educating children with autism. National Academy Press, Washington, DC

Perera H, Jeewandara KC, Seneviratne S, Guruge C (2016) Outcome of home-based early intervention for autism in Sri Lanka: follow-up of a cohort and comparison with a nonintervention group. Bio Med Res Int 2016:3284087. https://doi.org/10.1155/2016/3284087

Perry R, Cohen I, DeCarlo R (1995) Case study: deterioration, autism, and recovery in two siblings. J Am Acad Child Adolesc Psychiatry 34:232–237

Perrya A, Cummings A, Geier JD, Freeman NL, Hughes S, LaRose L, Managhan T, Reitzel JA, Williams J (2008) Effectiveness of intensive behavioral intervention in a large, community-based program. Res Autism Spectr Disord 2(4):621–642

Pierce K, Schreibman L (1995) Increasing complex social behaviors in children with autism: effects of peer-implemented pivotal response training. J Appl Behav Anal 28:285–295

Risley T, Hart B, Doke L (1972) Operant language development: the outline of a therapeutic technology. In: Schiefelbusch RL (ed) Language of the mentally retarded. University Park Press, Baltimore, MD, pp 107–123

Romanczyk RG (1996) Behavior analysis and assessment: the cornerstone to effectiveness. In: Maurice C, Green G, Luce SC (eds) Behavioral intervention for young children with autism: a manual for parents and profgessionals. Austin, TX, Pro-Ed, pp 195–217

Sallows GO, Graupner TD (2005) Intensive behavioral treatment of children with autism: four year outcome and predictors. Am J Ment Retard 110(6):417–438

Sarokoff RA, Taylor BA (2001) Teaching children with autism to engage in conversation exchanges: script fading with embedded textual stimuli. J Appl Behav Anal 34:81–84

Symes MD, Remington B, Brown T (2006) Early intensive intervention for children with autism: therapists' perspective on achieving procedural fidelity. Res Dev Disabil 27:30–42

Wacker DP, Steege MW, Northup J, Sasso G, Berg W, Reimers T et al (1990) A component analysis of functional communication training across three topographies of severe behavior problems. J Appl Behav Anal 23:417–429

Welterlin A, Turner-Brown LM, Harris S, Mesibov G, Delmolino L (2012) (2012). The home TEACCHing program for toddlers with autism. J Autism Dev Disord 42:1827–1835. https://doi.org/10.1007/s10803-011-1419-2

Wieder S, Greenspan S (2005) Can children with autism master the core deficits and become empathetic, creative, and reflective? J Dev Learn Disorders 9:1–15

Williams WS, Keonig K, Scahill L (2007) Social skills development in children with autism spectrum disorders: a review of the intervention research. J Autism Dev Disord 37:1858–1868. https://doi.org/10.1007/s10803-006-0320-x

Chapter 3
Role of Technology in Autism Intervention

3.1 Introduction

In the last chapter, I introduced you to the various dimensions of conventional intervention set at home, community centre, and school environment. Though this technique is powerful, yet there are several limitations related to availing specialized intervention services. For example, some of the potent barriers to gaining accessibility to such intervention are restricted availability of appropriately trained therapists, necessity of the caregiver to accompany the child needing specialized services, need to travel long distances for accessing such services, lack of appropriate data that can suggest the type of intervention that will work best for specific children (that is critical given the spectrum nature of autism with each child with autism being unique), exorbitant costs of one-on-one therapy sessions, etc. (Ganz 2007; Goodwin 2008). Given these limitations and the importance of offering early intervention services, investigators are now exploring the use of technology to develop platforms that possess the positive attributes of conventional intervention and can (1) cater to each child's need (i.e. individualized), (2) be cost-effective so that it is accessible to the public at large, (3) offer metrics that can quantify one's progress post intervention, (4) offer intensive intervention, etc. to address at least some of the core deficit areas characterizing autism (Goodwin 2008).

3.2 Advantages of Technology-Based Intervention Services

With increased prevalence and awareness of autism, there is a consensus that properly designed, individualized early behavioural and educational intervention services can be beneficial for both the children with autism and their families. Specifically, this can help in addressing at least some of the core social communication vulnerabilities commonly seen in individuals with autism (NRC 2001). There

© Springer Nature Switzerland AG 2020
U. Lahiri, *A Computational View of Autism*,
https://doi.org/10.1007/978-3-030-40237-2_3

is a large body of literature that have indicated the importance of technology in autism intervention. With technological progress and people becoming more technology-savvy, many investigators have shown the utility of using advanced interactive technologies.

For example, researchers have shown the applicability of technological solutions such as computer technology and robotic systems for offering assistive intervention platforms (Blocher and Picard 2002; Kozima et al. 2005; Parsons et al. 2004; Ploog et al. 2013). These studies have reported the positive contribution of technology towards autism intervention to address various aspects of one's social communication skills. Also, these platforms can hold promise in offering individualized intervention that can be potent to help these individuals to overcome some of the deficits adversely affecting their community lives. This, in turn, can help them to lead a productive community life. Here, I offer some of the advantages in the use of technology for intervention.

3.2.1 Improvement in Ability to Communicate

Children with autism often experience social communication-related milestones that manifest itself in terms of the difficulty to express their thoughts and communicate their needs. Such an experience can often be frustrating for both the child and his or her family. For example, if a child is thirsty and wants to drink water, but cannot express or communicate his need to another person such as a family member, then it might be annoying for the child. In such a case, the child might lose his composure and behave in ways that might be socially inappropriate. This can have cascading effects, such as the child might exhibit a tendency to cause self-injuries, might feel that his emotional needs are not satisfied, can cause him to be separated from the society, etc. In such cases, technology can offer them with an alternative platform to communicate their thoughts, emotions, etc. to their social partners.

Let us consider the picture-based communication modality using an iPad (e.g. AVAZ) used as an Augmented and Alternative Communication tool (Sankardas and Rajanahally 2017). The AVAZ has a graphical user interface that displays picture icons which can be selected by a child to communicate his needs and feelings. Also, the child can type the words so that his needs can be communicated to a social partner. For example, if a child is thirsty and wants to drink water, then the child can use this tool to select icons showing 'I', 'want', and 'water'. Then the tool can be used to offer an audio message corresponding to the child's need (based on the selected icons). Again, let us consider another example in which AVAZ can be used to carry out to-and-fro communication between a child and his or her social partner. One such scenario can be in which a child is found as less active in the morning. Thus, to find out the reason, the mother asks 'What has happened to you?' In response to the mother's question, the child can type the words 'I', 'am', 'not', and 'well' and the AVAZ says that out. Upon understanding that the child is not active because he is not feeling well, the mother might think of giving medicine to the child. In such a case, the mother might ask 'What is hurting you?' In response, the child might type 'stomach' followed by 'ache' that AVAZ speaks out. Thus, the mother can understand that her child is suffering from stomach ache and accordingly give the right medicine to her child.

3.2.2 Emotion Recognition

It is quite well known that children with autism are often characterized by deficits in picking up subtle cues from social communicators along with appropriate recipro-cation to emotional expressions. In conventional behavioural intervention, flashcard therapy is often used. Here, the children need to memorize the emotional expressions (shown through images on flashcards) that often becomes painstaking for these children (Lerman et al. 2004). Technological solutions can become handy in such cases as well. For example, researchers have reported the use of specialized eye glasses (using google glasses) to help children decode emotion by classifying emotional expressions such as happy, angry, sad, etc. (Washington et al. 2016; Voss et al. 2016). These researchers have demonstrated the use of google glasses in offering nearly real-time feedback on a social communicator's emotional expres-sion to the wearer that is the child with autism wearing the pair of glasses. The glasses have an outward facing camera that picks up the image of the face of a communicator and uses machine learning techniques to interpret various emotional expressions as demonstrated by the communicator. For computation, the researchers have used android phone integrated with the glasses. The feedback is offered in various modalities such as visual and auditory. The visual feedback can be in the form of text, colour, and an emoticon (as is preferred by the child) that appear on the glasses. The audio feedback is delivered as an audio message coupled with specific sounds. Additionally, these glasses have been integrated with eye tracking cameras that pick up the movement of the pupil (of the eye) of the child and offer information on whether the child had made eye contact with the social partner during the communication.

3.2.3 Assistance in Learning

Many children with autism are visual learners (Hodgdon 1999). Sometimes teaching using instructional mode delivered in a typical classroom setting may not work well for these children. In such cases, use of tablets and other mobile devices, computers, etc. that can make a visual presentation of facts can be helpful for these children to learn skills. For example, researchers such as Holt and Yuill (2017) have come up with a wifi-enabled dual tablet configuration that helps to develop awareness towards others, imitation and communication in children with learning disabilities. By using the dual tablet configuration, a child can play with his or her teacher or a peer. Here, the picture sequencing task was used. Pictures of activities were displayed in a randomized manner to the children. The players can choose a sequence of pictures using the dual tablet configuration. Again, researchers such as Sampath et al. (2012) have used tablets as an Augmentative and Alternative Communication tool for children with autism. This uses the concepts of Picture Exchange Communication System (PECS) that is commonly used for these children (Charlop-Christy et al. 2002). In this study, the participants were children with autism and they were mostly non-verbal. The database consisted of images of food items that were preferred by the child. For example, if there were few food items available in the house for breakfast, the mother would choose the pictures of the available items to be displayed on the tablet. Then the child was expected to choose from among these for her breakfast.

3.2.4   Intervention Cost

Conventional one-on-one therapy sessions require intense involvement from specially-trained therapists. Such services can be very expensive (Roddy and Neill 2018). Researchers such as Beuscher et al. (2014) have reported estimates of the annual cost of childhood autism to be £3.4 billion in the UK and US$66 billion in the USA. The cost of intervention increases with the age of the child. For adults, the estimated annual cost is about £31 billion and US$196 billion, respectively. Thus, such services might not be affordable for the public at large. Technology can serve as a complementary tool in the intervention process. With increased computational power and technological explosion, electronic gadgets have become cheaper and can often be accessed by the public. The technology-assisted learning requires one-time investment for setting it up and the child can be offered repeated exposure to the learning environment. Also, these technology-assisted tools can offer variations within the learning environment, thereby helping in the generalization of the skills learnt. Also, such variations can help in avoiding possible feeling of monotony among the children during the training process. Also, if a child achieves a certain level of proficiency in a task, the technology-assisted environment can adaptively increase the task difficulty to offer an increased challenge to the learners.

3.2.5   Quantitative Estimation of Affective States

With rapid technological progress, computers and robots can be easily augmented with extended functionalities such as sensing a child's looking pattern, behavioural manifestations, and other involuntary measures such as physiological signals (e.g. heart rate, blink rate, and pupillary dilation) that can offer estimates of a child's affective state while undergoing a technology-driven intervention. These subtle measures, though difficult to be picked up through observation, can be easily deciphered by technology to offer quantitative estimates of one's affective state. For example, on seeing a particular visual stimulus, a child with autism might feel happy that he cannot express and the emotional response can be manifested as changes in heart rate, blinking, etc. Since the child with autism has communication vulnerabilities that restrict the child from making an explicit expression of his/her emotions, tapping into other modalities such as physiology might be helpful. In such a case, the computer (say) that is presenting the visual task to the child can easily be interfaced with external peripheral devices that can sense the variation in the physiological parameters and identify the affective state of the child executing the task. Also, this information can offer valuable insights to the therapist regarding the physiological profile of the child along with quantitative estimates of the affective states of the child. In turn, the therapist can modify the intervention paradigm to better suit the child's abilities. Also with increased computational power, the computer can be programmed to autonomously decode the affective state of the child from the measured physiology and can be tuned to change the intervention so as to suit to the child's need.

3.2.6 Overcoming Resource Limitation

Often gaining access to specialized intervention services is difficult for the families of children with autism. This is particularly true in developing countries like India, where specialized services delivered by trained interventionists are often located in selected pockets of the urban community. Often the parents have to commute long distances with their child to avail specialized services. The technology-based intervention platforms can serve as a complementary tool. With technology-based solutions, some of the intervention can be done in the homes with caregivers administering the intervention. Additionally, these devices often become useful to the therapists. Specifically, this can enable a therapist to administer intervention for a number of children at the same time with variations in the training delivery (possible with technology) based on individualized requirements. In other words, this can help address the lack of availability of adequately trained therapists coupled with reduced waiting time for the child and his or her family in accessing the intervention services.

3.2.7 Versatility in the Training Environment

It is known that children with autism find it difficult to generalize the learned skills across different social situations. For example, let us consider a hypothetical situation in which a child is taught the skill of navigating within a social gathering such as at a festival while following social etiquettes. The child can be expected to transfer the knowledge gained in such a situation to another situation, e.g. a restaurant environment (say) while navigating through it. However, the child may experience difficulties in generalizing across situations. This lays the importance on offering varying situations to the child during skill training. Again, offering variations in the training scenarios might make skill training interesting to the children. Thus, it is useful to have variations in the skill training environments. Getting to offer variations within the clinician's therapeutic setting is not always feasible. In such a case, technology can have a role to play. In fact, with progress in Human Computer Interaction, designers are now empowered to develop skill training environments with variations. Specifically, recently, researchers have been using computer-based environment with Virtual Reality (VR) that can project various contexts related to learning of specific skills to the children with autism.

3.2.8   Controllability

It is an established fact that children with autism often become uncomfortable in social situations. This can be partly attributed to the fact that real-life social settings are often complex, dynamic, etc. Thus, a child with autism being exposed to such a scenario might find it difficult to cope up with the complex social needs. This might adversely affect the child's ability to learn skills. In such a case, if the complexity of the social scenario can be controlled, then this can help in scaffolded skill learning. For example, let us consider a restaurant environment and the child is to be taught the art of navigating within such a social scene, order food, pay for the food, find a place to sit, etc. while following social etiquettes. Exposing the child to a busy restaurant environment towards the very beginning of the training might not work for the child. In turn, training can be imparted by introducing the child to restaurant environments with gradually increasing complexity. In other words, the level of complexity can be controlled. For example, at first the child can be introduced to a restaurant environment that is sparsely populated with most of the tables as empty. Thus, the child is taught how to move between the tables and take his seat at one of the empty tables. In case, he wants to sit at a table that is partially occupied, it would be a good social practice to ask the occupant sitting at the table to know if the other empty seats (at the table) are meant for someone else known to that occupant. Subsequently, the child can be exposed to a restaurant environment that is populated. Since the child has learned the social etiquettes that one can expect of him while occupying a seat, the child will face less difficulty in applying the knowledge learnt, thereby allowing him to find a seat at the restaurant. Now offering such scenes to the child in real-life settings might be difficult. The technology can be used to offer such controlled settings. For example, computer-based Virtual Reality situations with controlled levels of complexity can be easily designed and projected in front of the child. Once the child becomes accustomed to such settings, the child can be exposed to real-life restaurant environments.

3.2.9   Individualization

Autism being a spectrum disorder, each child with autism is unique. Thus, for effective skill learning, the training scenarios need to be preferably individualized that are tuned to the child's specific needs. For example, there can be different modes of learning such as verbal, visual, kinesthetic, etc. that can be preferred by a child. A child with low-functioning autism might face difficulties with motor activities. For such a child, the skill training environment projected by a computer-based platform can use the audio-visual mode instead of kinaesthetic mode of communication. Also, the child can be expected to interact with the computer-based social setting by using eye movement or by speaking out. With technological progress, computers can be easily integrated with external peripherals such as eye trackers that can track one's eye movement while viewing a social scene. Also, there have been good audio decoders that can decipher one's verbal prompt and convey that to the computer-based task environment. However, if the child with autism is high functioning, he might prefer to undertake an interactive gaming while conveying his choices to the computing medium through physical contact that is touching the computer screen presenting the visual stimulus. In such a case, added to the audio-visual modalities, the designer might add the element of kinaesthetics to the task engine used to project a skill training scenario in front of the child. This can be easily achieved through the use of technology.

3.2.10   Scalability

As already narrated before, offering training scenarios with controlled levels of challenge might be beneficial for a child with autism particularly at the initial stages of skill learning. Thus, the training environment must possess scalability. For example, exposing a child to a shopping mall with gradually increasing levels of complexity might need one to project scenes from the shopping mall with mild, moderate, and high levels of crowd at the different stalls inside the shopping mall. Getting such variations within a real-life social setting, particularly at the therapist's clinic, might be difficult. In such a case, technology can offer a viable alternative. For example, using Virtual Reality, one can project scenes from a shopping mall on a computer screen, with the amount of crowd being easily scaled up based on the training need. Again, let us consider that a child is taught the steps needed to cross a road. In such a case, technology can be used to scale up the road scenes with gradually increasing traffic, thereby slowly increasing the difficulty of the skill learning environment.

3.2.11 Safety

Use of technology to teach skills to the children with autism often serves to present training scenarios that can guarantee the safety of the child. For example, let us consider a hypothetical scenario in which a child with autism is exposed to a park environment. Now a child possessing deficit in social communication might reciprocate in ways that are not appropriate for establishing fluid communication with a social communicator, say another child in the park. In such a case, the child with autism might not be handled properly by the other children in the park. Specifically, due to the inappropriate disposition, the child with autism might be rebuked that in turn further deters the child from entering into social conversation in future. Instead, the child can be given tips on handling social scenarios in a park environment by offering technology-based gaming scenarios to the child for skill training before exposing him to the actual park environment. The Virtual Reality-based games can be designed to project various park environments coupled with simulated agents that can serve as facilitators, giving important information to the child if the child commits mistakes while interacting with the social partners. With simulated platform, a child can be free to make mistakes without experiencing any negative consequences. In turn, the technology-assisted skill training platform can offer a safe learning environment for a child.

3.3 Technology-based Applications to Address Deficits

With technological explosion, children of the present day are becoming more conversant with the use of technology. Given this fact, researchers have been pondering on ways to harness this attraction to the use of technology to promote skill learning among the children. In the following sections, I will be presenting the use of technology such as robots and computers to address skill deficits experienced by children with ASD.

3.3.1 Robotic Technology: Addressing Skill Deficits

The technological advancement in the realm of robotics has led to the advent of autonomous robotic systems that have now become part and parcel of our daily lives. Service robots in homes for the elderly, factory, restaurants, etc. are slowly moving towards being a reality. These robots might be used for security purposes, vacuum cleaning of floors, interacting with children in games, etc. While harnessing the technological progress, investigators are trying to make the Human Robot Interaction (HRI) become more natural and meaningful. This is possible by offering emotional intelligence to robots while utilizing concepts of artificial intelligence.

Research shows increased acceptance of robots by children with autism and there is evidence from literature that shows the robots can be potentially used for skill learning (Robins et al. 2004). The acceptance of robots by children with autism can be partially attributed to the fact that the robot offers a medium whose behaviour can be predicted and can be easily understood by the children. While the presence of a robot in a learning environment offers a 3D embodiment, it can be designed in ways that possesses reduced complexity in its appearance unlike that of the real-life social communicators. For example, one can design a toy-like robot. Also, the tone, pitch, etc. of the robot's voice can be designed with limited variations that can be less confusing for the children with autism. Researchers have reported that children with autism interact with robots, express concern for them and focus on them in ways that are often similar to their typically developing peers (Duquette et al. 2007). There is a rich history of literature that has reported the use of robots in various applications some of which are listed below.

3.3.1.1 Robots for Emotion-related Skill Learning

Researchers have been using technology to design robots that can display emotions by showing facial expressions, gesture, etc. similar to that exhibited by human beings. Of course, the manner and the intensity of the emotional expressions can be different and depends on the designer. One of the examples is the Pong robot developed by the IBM group (Haritaoglu et al. 2001). This robot can track the face of a user, recognize changes in facial emotional expression and can mimic the face of a user.

Others are Kismet and Leonardo developed by MIT (Breazeal 2000; Hoffman and Breazeal 2004) to demonstrate social intelligence that is important for skill learning by children with autism. Specifically, for a robot to behave like a (human) teammate, the robot needs to have the capability to recognize what an individual is doing and understand the inherent intention of the partner while doing the task. The robot Leonardo has been designed with such a capability (Hoffman and Breazeal 2004) giving rise to the term human–robot collaboration instead of human–robot interaction. To achieve this, the robot is equipped with visual, auditory, and proprioceptive sensory inputs so as to facilitate parent–child interaction. The social robot Leonardo has been equipped with visual tracking system and programs based on infant psychology.

Another example is the ATR's (Japan) Robovie-IIS (Kanda et al. 2002). Researchers have reported Robovie's application as a museum guide who can autonomously take the children around a museum while informing them on the different exhibits (Shiomi et al. 2006). Again, robots equipped with emotional intelligence have also reached the toy industry. One of the socially interactive robotic toys was the robot dog AIBO. This robot demonstrated ability to learn new behaviours based on interaction with humans. Researchers have reported that the AIBO was accepted by children with autism during play (Stanton et al. 2008).

Another robot KASPAR has been reported to be able to display different facial emotional expressions (Blow et al. 2006). Here, the researchers have worked on the finer aspects of facial emotional expression. For example, when KASPAR smiled, the smile was not only shown in the mouth region. Instead, to make it more realistic, smiling of the robot was accompanied by its cheeks being raised along with a narrowing of its eyes. This robot was accepted by the children with autism who could focus on KASPAR's face without displaying any anxiety, commonly experienced by these children when they interact with social partners (humans).

3.3.1.2   Robots for Teaching Vocabulary

Use of relevant language is important for appropriate reciprocation during social communication. Such a skill is generally intact in typically developing children. In fact, children between 1.5 years and 2 years display a rapid spurt in vocabulary. A 2-year toddler can often be seen to make use of vocabulary in different contexts (Mody and Belliveau 2013). Often, a typically developing child uses language to start social communication (Wetherby 1986). However, a child with autism uses language to control her environment, e.g. to demand for what she wants or to protest. These children might often suffer from apraxia or oral-motor deficits that can adversely affect their capability to communicate (Mody and Belliveau 2013). This is also evident in the pre-verbal stage of development in which a child with autism has deficits in the use of symbolic language such as pointing towards an object of interest. Instead the child might physically move another's hand to point towards an object of interest. This adversely affected developmental process is often manifested in terms of delayed or impaired language abilities at an early age (Luyster et al. 2008) of a child with autism.

Robot-assisted techniques have been reported to be potent in imparting such skills in children with ASD. Researchers have shown that robots can be used to improve vocabulary of toddlers. Specifically, researchers have been exploring the applicability of robots in education, even in elementary schools (Lee et al. 2011; Han et al. 2008). It has been also found that children prefer interacting with robots (Tanaka and Matsuzoe 2012). The majority of the educational robots that have been designed so far have been mostly for enacting the role of a teacher or a caregiver. Thus, the robot can be used to teach the child using two modalities. One modality can be in which the child is asked to teach the robot that in turn helps the child to learn. In another case, the robot is used to teach the child. For example, in the first case, the parents might ask the child to teach a topic to a robot. First when the child teaches the robot, the robot does not appear to understand the topic being taught. In due course, the robot appears to learn the topic on multiple instructions given by the child. In this process, the child also learns (Tanaka and Matsuzoe 2012). In the latter case, robots can be used to teach topics such as vocabulary to children with autism. For example, researchers such as Alemia and Mahboub (2016) have shown the use of robot-assisted learning to teach English-language vocabulary words to non-English-speaking children with autism. Here, the researchers used a Nao robot. This is a 3D humanoid robot with up to 25 degrees of freedom. It can demonstrate gestures, walk, sit down, stand, speak, etc. For example, one of the applications deal with teaching English vocabulary in which the children are expected to speak in English if they would like to interact with the robot. Since the children generally like interacting with the robot, they show a desire to speak in English to carry on the conversation with the robot. It can start with introducing each other followed by shaking hands.

One of the research studies have shown an improvement of ~27% in mastering target words by toddlers, 18–24 months in age compared to a matched set of control words when training was facilitated by a robot (Movellan et al. 2009). Thus, robots can be used to effectively contribute to early childhood education, even for children with autism.

3.3.1.3 Robots for Teaching Imitation and Turn-Taking

Imitation is a mechanism that can be employed for learning appropriate behaviour (Scassellati et al. 2012) that is important for carrying out lucid social communication. Generally, in typically developing children, the ability to imitate appears early in age (Meltzoff and Moore 1977) and has been reported to be important in developing cognitive and social behaviours such as using language, demonstrating joint attention, etc. (Rogers and Pennington 1991). For example, in early face-to-face interactions, typically developing infants tend to demonstrate imitation either by repeating the words said or by imitating emotional expressions while interacting with their adult partners. One's ability to imitate leads to two major functions, namely learning function and social function (Ingersoll 2008). The learning function refers to that in which a child can learn new skills and knowledge. On the other hand, the social function refers to the ability of a child to be engaged socially and emotionally with a social partner. Another important aspect is the reciprocal imitation that becomes crucial in early interactions. Such a skill can help one to build social linkage with his or her communicators (Nadel et al. 1999). Children with autism often find it difficult in imitating actions such as gestures of social communicators (Williams et al. 2004a, b). A longitudinal study has shown that gestural imitation and language development can be highly correlated in children with autism (Stone et al. 1997).

Thus, inclusion of games in an intervention that focus on usage of imitation and turn-taking skills is important since this can lead to an improvement in one's body awareness and sense of self, creativity, etc. (Payne 1990). Researchers have reported that using imitation in game scenarios can help to develop social interaction skills in the children with autism (Costonis 1978; Adler 1968). Researchers also have shown the potential of using robot-assisted skill learning to impart various skills such as imitation, turn-taking, etc. For example, interactive autonomous robots (such as in the AURORA project) can engage children with autism in imitation games to administer training in various aspects of human–human interaction through the use of human–robot interaction (Dautenhahn and Werry 2004). In this, the researchers use a robot named Kaspar that is a child-sized 3D humanoid robot. This robot has

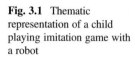

Fig. 3.1 Thematic representation of a child playing imitation game with a robot

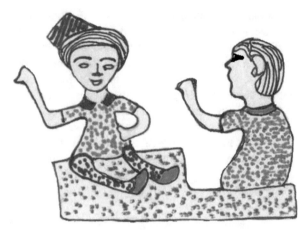

15 degrees of freedom in its head and neck, arms and torso. The robot can be used to teach skills to a child using imitation (Fig. 3.1).

During intervention, the games can be designed to facilitate in imparting imitation skills in children with autism either in a structured manner or spontaneously. In the structured approach, the children are encouraged by a robot performing animations to imitate its actions through meaningful tasks and interactive play (Ferrari et al. 2009). The play was designed to help children to learn turn-taking, follow rules and pay respect to the opinions of social partners in the play. Specifically, these were designed as games with exercise, assembly, symbols, and rules. While using the spontaneous approach, the intervention can be delivered in the form of a game in which both the child and the robot imitate each other's actions (Kozima et al. 2007). The game can be designed to go a step further by incorporating triadic actions involving a therapist, the robot and the child to impart skills related to turn-taking and sharing. The idea was that, once the dyadic interaction (between the child and robot) was established, then the child can be exposed to a triadic interaction in which there can be interaction among the child, a robot and another human being.

3.3.1.4 Robot to Administer Joint Attention Skill Training

Joint attention (JA) skills are considered to be one of the fundamental building blocks of the social communication. Joint attention has been broadly defined in terms of responding to joint attention (RJA) and initiating joint attention (IJA) (Mundy and Newell 2007). The RJA occurs when an individual follows the cue delivered by a social partner and attends to a stimulus. The IJA refers to the initiation of an intentional cuing to get the attention of another individual towards a stimulus. For effective social communication, added to the IJA, one needs to exhibit appropriate reciprocation through demonstration of RJA. Thus, if a social partner has initiated a task through cuing while prompting towards a target of interest, the RJA

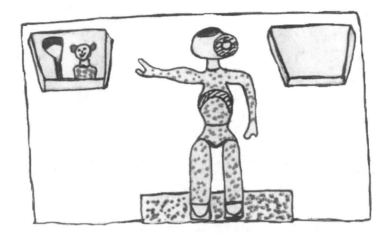

Fig. 3.2   Thematic representation of a robot administering JA task

can be considered as 'Looking where someone else is looking' (Sigman et al. 1995). Again, the JA also refers to a triadic exchange in which a child coordinates his or her gaze between his or her social partner and a target of interest. In conventional intervention, a therapist administers JA skill training while prompting a child through the use of cues such as looking, finger pointing, etc. towards a target of interest.

Children with autism are often characterized by deficits in JA skills (Mundy and Neal 2000; Poon et al. 2011). Motivated by this, researchers such as Bekele et al. (2013) have deployed robots to administer JA skill learning among children with autism while using multiple levels of prompting in an individualized manner. Here, the researchers have developed an Adaptive Robot-mediated Autism Intervention Architecture wherein a humanoid robot works in coordination with a network of spatially distributed cameras and display monitors to enable dynamic closed-loop interaction with a participant while imparting JA skill learning. Specifically, as shown in Fig. 3.2, a robot prompted a child to look towards monitors kept on the walls of a study room while administering JA tasks. The prompting was delivered though the demonstration of head turn, pointing gesture coupled with audio messages such as 'look at that'. If the child was able to respond to the JA task immediately after the first prompting such as a head turn towards the monitor of interest, then the robot rewarded the child by saying 'good job'. In case, the child was not able to complete the JA task, the robot increased the prompting by raising a pointed finger along with head turn as the prompting cue. As can be seen from Fig. 3.2, the robot has turned its head along with finger pointing (with a raised arm) towards its right to point towards the monitor kept on a wall on its right side. Thus, the robot was empowered to deliver hierarchically increasing prompts based on whether the child was capable of responding to the JA task. In certain cases, the system was capable of rewarding the child by playing videos of favourite cartoons on the target monitors towards which the child was prompted to look.

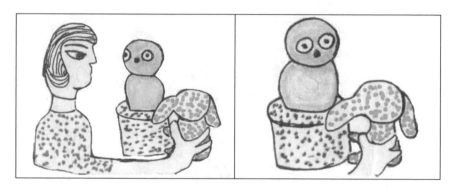

Fig. 3.3 Thematic representation of Keepon robot administering JA task

Again, investigators have used a robot called Keepon and remotely configured it to direct its eye gaze to look towards the child or towards a target of interest with an aim to prompt the child to look towards the cued target to administer a joint attention task (Kozima and Nakagawa 2006). Figure 3.3 shows a thematic representation of such a robot participating in the JA task while shifting its gaze from a participant towards a toy. The moment a child fixated on the target that was cued by Keepon in the JA task, Keepon would display animation such as rocking to indicate its excitement that in turn also served to encourage the child to interact with it.

Researchers from Japan have also used robots for autonomously administering goal-directed JA tasks while deciphering the intention of a child with autism (De Silva et al. 2009). In this, a child with autism was expected to respond to a finger pointing gesture issued by the robot while establishing JA. The task ran with a robot prompting towards an object of interest kept in front of the child and the robot. Initially, if required, the teacher helped the child in establishing the JA. If the child was able to pick up the cuing prompt delivered by the robot, then the robot displayed a joyful motion that served as a reward for the child. The computing platform associated with the robot kept a track of the time taken by the child to look towards the prompted target. If the JA was established, the robot invited the child to participate in another task while prompting towards a different object.

3.3.2 Computer-Based Technology: Addressing Skill Deficits

While contribution of robots in skill learning for children with autism is noteworthy, nowadays computers are getting a strong foothold in the area of autism intervention. With technological progress, computers have become part and parcel of our daily lives. Additionally, there had been growth in the area of computing power along with expansion in hardware capabilities achieved by augmenting the computational framework with external peripheral devices. Thus, computers have intruded the realm of entertainment and education. Also, with recent discoveries in the area of rich graphics, nowadays, computers can display graphical user interfaces that can be programmed to appear as colourful and realistic to which a child can easily relate himself or herself. Thus, imparting skills in children through the use of computers had become cost-effective, user-friendly, and motivating. As a result, computers find their place in homes, schools, and intervention clinics, often serving as a complementary tool in the hands of the trainer. Again computer-based training modules can be easily individualized so as to suit one's requirement. This may not be feasible in classroom teaching with a large number of students where instructions are systematically delivered to the students following certain framework. However, this traditional classroom setting may not work for all children such as children with autism. Autism being a spectrum disorder, each child is unique and might necessitate modification of the delivery pattern so as to suit to the child's specific need.

Computer-based instruction (Ramdoss et al. 2012) that can be tuned to offer educational materials in an individualized manner can serve as a complementary platform to classroom teaching. In fact, this can augment the ability of the trainer to offer individualized instructions for skill learning in non-traditional domains, such as social and emotional skill learning based on the cognitive functioning of the students (Whalen et al. 2010). Moreover, computers can offer a controlled environment where distractions can be minimized, thereby helping the students with autism to be attentive to feedback and prompts delivered by the computer (Williams et al. 2002). There is also the flip side of the coin where computer-based instruction can have its own limitations. Excessive use of computer might alienate the students from reality, thereby adversely affecting the social interaction skills in individuals with autism (Powell 1996). Thus, care needs to be taken while monitoring the progress of the child in the computer-assisted skill learning. In turn, one can easily move from a dyadic communication between the child and the computer to a triadic communication involving the child, the computer and a peer or a caregiver. Given the benefits of using computers, such a platform has been applied to both typically developing individuals (Inan et al. 2010) and individuals with autism (Hetzroni and Shalem 2005). The literature review indicates the applicability of computer-based intervention in imparting skill learning in the areas of communication (Ramdoss et al. 2011a), literacy (Ramdoss et al. 2011b), spelling (Vedora and Stromer 2007), and a host of other areas for individuals with autism. Added to skill training in the area of academics, computer-assisted training has shown promise in the areas of imitation, false belief and joint attention.

With technological progress and increase in computational power, delivering tailored skill training to the target group is now a reality. Also, users have become computer-savvy. Additionally, computer-assisted training can be offered in a cost-effective manner, thereby making it easily accessible to the various stakeholders even in countries with developing economies.

3.3.2.1 Computer for Teaching Communication Skill

Children with autism are often characterized by deficits in communication skills (APA 2000) related to initiation of conversation, imitating spoken sentences, etc.

This is one of the earliest symptoms demonstrated by these children (Eigsti et al. 2007). Such deficits in communication skills might make it difficult for these children to exchange thoughts with social partners. Thus, this can have cascading effects on these children that is marked by behavioural disorders in later stages with subsequent reduction in their enrollment in traditional schools and inclusion in the community (Sigafoos et al. 2006). To address such deficits, children with autism are often referred to intervention centres. Intervention aimed at training the children in communication skills is often complex, necessitating long hours of one-on-one therapy sessions between the child and a therapist with the aim of delivering individualized training that can suit one's need. Then only training can be effective in imparting skills to the child. In such a scenario, the use of computers can become important. This is because, computers can be easily programmed to flexibly simulate varying situations pivoted on different aspects of social communication for delivering individualized communication skill training to these children.

There is a rich history of literature that provides evidence of the potential of computers to impart communication skill-related training focused on (1) vocabulary, (2) vocal imitation with regard to (a) imitation of syllables and (b) framing of sentences, (3) initiation of conversation, and (4) ability to appropriately reciprocate.

3.3.2.1.1 Computer for Teaching Vocabulary Words

Research has shown the potential of computer-based instruction to teach vocabulary words to these children. This can serve to improve one's language receptive skills (Massaro and Bosseler 2006). During social communication, apart from listening to a voice, looking towards the movement of the lips, face, jaws, etc. also become useful. The researchers have used a Vocabulary Wizard that appears as an animated head on the computer screen with accurate auditory and visible speech capability. Figure 3.4 shows a thematic representation of such a face used by the researchers. The graphical user interface could display pictures and deliver spoken words. The animated head was able to talk and the audio version of the words was delivered using text-to-speech conversion programs. Additionally, images of the vocabulary words used were displayed. The Wizard started by narrating a short description for each vocabulary word while the corresponding image was displayed on the computer screen. For example, if the images of the telescope, broom, tool kit, etc. were displayed on the screen and the animated head said 'one can see with this device', then a child was expected to choose the telescope. Again, if the head said that 'you sweep with this', then the child was expected to choose the broom. This was administered through two phases. First was the vocabulary acquisition phase. This was followed by the vocabulary testing phase. The system gave feedback on how the child had performed in the picture-word mapping task by offering reward as a reinforcer. For example, if the child made a right choice, then a happy emoticon was displayed on the screen as a reinforcer.

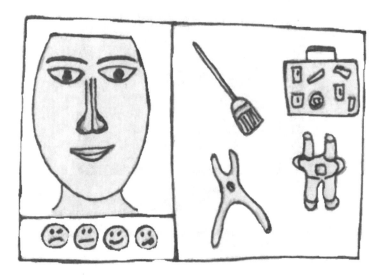

Fig. 3.4 Thematic representation of a Vocabulary Wizard with objects

3.3.2.1.2   Computer for Teaching Vocal Imitation and Imitation of Syllables

Research shows that almost one-thirds of the children with autism fail to use spoken words and instead they use alternate non-verbal communication modes, such as using hand signs, picture cards, etc. (Quill 1997). Also, most of the non-verbal children exhibit minimal vocal imitation with reduced skills to imitate sounds (Stone et al. 1990). However, these children often show a better or even normal ability to undertake the visual discrimination task. This is evident from their capability of solving puzzles and remembering locations (Siegel et al., 1996). This fact motivated investigators to use computer-generated visual feedback to help these children in the area of vocalization. As far as the vocal imitation is concerned, the computer-based instruction has shown promise in imparting training while helping a child in imitation of syllables (Bernard-Opitz et al. 1999). Researchers such as Colby (1973) have used computers to impart speech training in these children. For example, if a child pressed the letter 'H' on a keyboard, then the letter 'H' would appear on the screen accompanied by a voice that pronounced 'H'. Also, the child was exposed to tasks of varying difficulty levels. For example, when the child pressed 'H' on the keyboard, a horse appeared on the screen (Fig. 3.5 shows an example) that ran across the screen while the child could hear the sound of its hoofs.

While imitating syllables, importance of loudness and accuracy of pronunciation needs to be emphasized. For imparting training on imitation of syllables, computer-based modules are designed to improve one's awareness to sound, loudness, vowel accuracy, etc. (Bernard-Opitz et al. 1999). To make these training modules interesting, these researchers have programmed visual feedback (displayed on the computer monitor) in response to the performed task. For example, to give a feedback on the

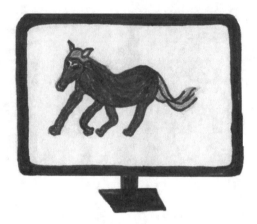

Fig. 3.5 A running horse appearing on a computer screen while 'H' is pressed on the keyboard

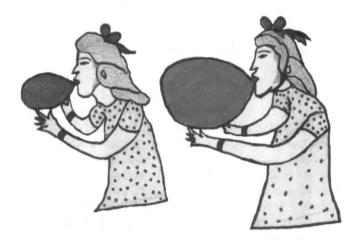

Fig. 3.6 Thematic representation of the size of a blown balloon depending on the loudness level being (**a**) low and (**b**) high (as a pictorial representation of the example)

loudness level, the computer-based system offered different types of visual imagery such as blowing a balloon as a function of loudness. Figure 3.6 shows a thematic representation of such a feedback. Again, feedback can be tuned to address both the volume and the correctness of the pronunciation. For example, Bernard-Opitz et al. (1999) had used the jumping of a monkey from a base station while moving up a tree as a feedback if the vowels were pronounced audibly and correctly. Figure 3.7 shows a thematic representation of such a feedback.

Fig. 3.7 Thematic
representation of a monkey
climbing up a tree (as a
pictorial representation of
the example)

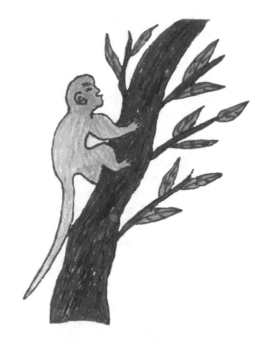

Fig. 3.8 Cat sitting on a
mat (as a pictorial
representation of the
example)

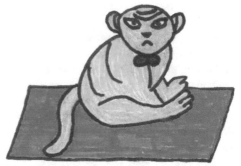

3.3.2.1.3   Computer for Teaching the Skill to Frame Sentences

Researchers (Heimann et al. 1995) have designed a computer-based training platform that facilitated a child to incrementally learn how to make sentences. This
training consisted of learning individual words accompanied with relevant imagery,
followed by testing a child on whether he or she has mastered the art of using single
words that in turn was followed by knitting the words to form sentences using noun-
verb-noun complexes along with visual animation, etc.

For example, let us consider a sentence creation using two nouns such as 'the cat'
and 'the mat' and one verb such as 'sits'. If a child chose the proper nouns and verb
to frame a sentence 'The cat sits on the mat', then the system offered a pictorial
representation of a cat sitting on the mat that can be useful for the visual learners.
Figure 3.8 shows an example of a pictorial representation of such a feedback. Again,

in the testing phase, the pictorial presentation of the noun-verb-noun complex was shown to the child and the child was expected to frame the sentence describing the display.

3.3.2.1.4   Computer for Teaching Initiation and Reciprocation During Social Conversation

Ability to initiate and respond to social greetings is crucial for one's seamless integration with the social community. Children with autism often face difficulties in initiating and responding to social greetings adversely affecting their social lives. This deficit can be possibly attributed to their limited ability to understand social conventions and difficulty in comprehending another's perspective (Harris et al. 1990). Since these children are often good visual learners, research has shown that observation-based learning of social models can be beneficial for them in learning appropriate social behaviours (Bandura et al. 1961). Specifically, observation of typically developing peers interacting in real-life social settings has been reported to be a powerful tool for teaching appropriate social behaviour and also in encouraging generalization (Chandler et al. 1992; Elksnin and Elksnin 1998). Thus, attempts had been made in developing social skills curricula pivoted on various social skills such as conversation skills (Ogeltree and Fischer 1995), greetings (Charlop-Christy et al. 2000), responding to others during social interaction (Norris and Dattilo 1999), etc. One of the difficulties in developing such curricula is design of variations in the social settings that might take a toll on the resources. Video-based instruction can offer an easy alternative in which variations in settings can be projected through simulation of real-life social interactions. This in turn can help in promoting generalization.

Computer-based instruction can be potent to improve one's ability to initiate a social conversation (Simpson et al. 2004). These investigators have developed videos of typically developing children sharing things with others, complying with the instructions of the teacher and adhering to the etiquettes by using social greetings. The videos were then presented to the learners with autism. While the individuals with autism observed the videos, the researchers recorded the manner in which the learners behaved in terms of initiating social conversation. Again, an ability to reciprocate appropriately to questions asked by a social partner is important for establishing effective two-way social communication. Computer-based instruction shows promise in imparting skills related to reciprocation in social communication (Parsons and La Sorte 1993) in individuals with autism.

3.3.2.2   Computer for Imparting Literacy Skills

Often, individuals with autism face milestones in learning symbols and communicating academic concepts (Ramdoss et al. 2011b). One of the most popular Augmentative and Alternative Communication systems that tends to teach symbols to children with autism is the Picture Exchange Communication System (PECS) (Bondy and Frost 1994). Such pictorial representation of symbols can be beneficial for children with autism having little to no speech capability (Preston and Carter 2009).

Computers can be used to impart literacy skills since this medium can offer a visual presentation of the instructions that is generally well-received by the children with autism who are often reported to be visual learners (Whalen et al. 2010). While imparting literacy skills, researchers have used computers to help them learn alphabets (Travers et al. 2011), improve ability to construct sentences (Basil and Reyes 2003), build phonological awareness (Tjus et al. 1998), read (Basil and Reyes 2003), and use expressive (Whalen et al. 2010) and receptive (Whalen et al. 2010) language.

3.3.2.2.1   Computer for Teaching Alphabets

One's ability to read is important for achieving independence, earning livelihood and enjoying quality community life (Education for all (EFA) 2005). As a prerequisite to such an ability one must be aware of alphabets. Researchers have shown the potential of computer-based training to impart knowledge of alphabets, even in preschool children with autism (Travers et al. 2011). For example, while teaching the alphabet 'H', computer-based training can expose a child to a visual schedule with different words (such as House) associated with the alphabet 'H' along with a brief description on certain specifics (such as rooms, size). All of these can be accompanied with relevant visual imagery. Figure 3.9 shows an example.

3.3.2.2.2   Computer for Developing Phonological Awareness

Phonological awareness refers to awareness towards the syllables and phonemes within words (Gillon 2004). The development of phonological awareness is important for decoding words (Miniscalcoa and Sandberg 2010). Research has shown a

Fig. 3.9 Use of visual imagery to teach the alphabet 'H' (as a pictorial representation of the example)

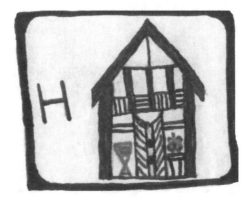

strong connection between language acquisition and phonological awareness (Magnusson and Naucle 1993). Many children with autism possess deficit in phonemic awareness (Vacca 2007).

Research has shown targeted sight-word intervention to be beneficial for these children (Gabig 2010). For developing phonological awareness, the investigators (Tjus et al. 1998) introduced the children with autism to the linkages among text, speech, and animation. These researchers used images with text that were displayed on the computer screen. When a learner picked up the texts to construct a sentence, then the system delivered an audio presentation of the generated sentence accompanied by a visual display of the animation to describe the sentence.

3.3.2.2.3 Computer for Developing Skills in Reading and in Use of Expressive Language

Researchers such as Basil and Reyes (Basil and Reyes 2003) have used computer to improve reading skills in children with autism. The children were required to select a word or group of words of varying complexity marked by the use of nouns, verbs, prepositions, etc. while interacting with a computer. Subsequently, the computer reads out the sentence followed by a visual presentation of a situation to depict the created sentence. Here, the researchers have used lessons that emphasize on learning noun-verb-noun complexes. To explain the concept behind the task, let us consider text, such as 'the gorilla', 'puts', 'the bowl', and 'the cat's table' along with prepositions such as 'on'. In this case, the children were expected to select the words and arrange these as 'the gorilla' 'puts' 'the bowl' 'on' 'the cat's table'. This is followed by a presentation of a visual stimulus. Figure 3.10 shows a thematic presentation.

There is evidence from literature that shows videos of environments and model displaying a target behaviour can be beneficial for children with autism to learn basics on behaviour (Nikopoulous and Keenan 2004) and also reducing problematic behaviours (Schreibman et al. 2000). Researchers such as Whalen et al. (2010) have

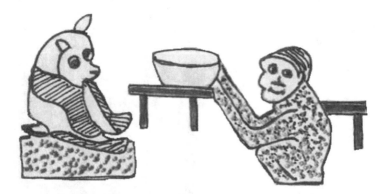

Fig. 3.10 Thematic presentation of a gorilla putting a bowl on the cat's table

used computer-based environment called as TeachTown that aimed to train a child on basics of behaviour. The TeachTown used the concepts of Applied Behaviour Analysis. This offered training in various domains, such as adaptive behaviour, cognitive skills, language, mathematics, social emotional learning, etc. This offered many examples to help children generalize the learnt skills. These researchers (Whalen et al. 2010) have reported that exposure to such an environment can contribute to a child's increased use of expressive language and reduced use of inappropriate language, even in situations outside the computer environment indicating the potential of computer-based training.

3.3.2.3   Computer for Teaching Spelling

Ability to write words in sentences with correct spelling can enable one to communicate properly with the literate world. Thus, learning to use correct spelling while writing sentences to express one's thought is an important part of the educational process (Heron et al. 1991). Researchers have reported that computers can be effectively used to teach a child the art of using correct spelling during writing, particularly for children with developmental disabilities (Vedora and Stromer 2007). Also, learning of spelling using computers has been shown to improve one's writing even outside the computing environment. For example, Stromer et al. (1996) have reported that children with autism who were taught spelling using computers were able to write correctly on index cards.

In the work by Vedora and Stromer (2007), the researchers exposed students with autism to computer-based anagram spelling task. In this, letters randomly appeared in the choice area. The student was expected to choose the letters in the correct order from the choice area by touching on the letters. Subsequently, these letters were populated in the construction area. If the learner's response was correct, then the computer made a flashing display. Post their computer-assisted learning, they were tested by asking them to write the correct spelling to check whether they have been able to learn the spelling.

Again, computer-based video models can be used for teaching spelling to children with autism. In a study by Kinney et al. (2003), the researchers asked the children to use their previously learnt consonants and word endings to formulate words. For example, use 'b' and 'at' to construct 'bat'. In the study by Kinney et al., the video was formed by focusing the camera on one author saying the second author to write a particular word. This was followed by the second author writing the targeted word with the camera focusing on the word being written. Finally, the written word was spoken out. Also, in another part of the study, a process called matrix training was used. In this, children were taught a subset of words in a matrix. Investigators showed that such technique was potent to enable the children to use correct spelling of other words, through recombinative generation (Mueller et al. 2000).

3.3.2.4   Computer for Teaching Social Communication Skills

Apart from conventional intervention techniques used for addressing the social communication deficit of the children with autism, computer-assisted training can offer a complementary platform. While leveraging on the visual learning capability of children with autism, researchers have proposed a combined effect of three strategies such as social stories, video modelling and computer-assisted instruction to be powerful in teaching social communication skills to these children (Sansosti and Powell-Smith 2008).

Social stories can be used to present contexts using imagery and text (Gray 1998) so as to understand a child's perspective to social situations. A social story can be useful to offer a description of a social situation, having agents appearing as social communicators and the thoughts of communicators, etc. Again, social stories can be formed in a way so as to offer suggestive actions that can facilitate a child to learn appropriate reciprocating mechanisms while dealing with such a situation. Instead of direct instruction, the social stories can offer detailed explanations so that one can understand and interpret what is expected in a particular situation (Ivey et al. 2004). Again, social stories have been shown to impart various skills in a child such as greeting skills and also the art of sharing toys with a social partner (Swaggart et al. 1995), reducing inappropriate behaviour (Crozier and Tincani 2005), increased demonstration of positive behaviour that is socially relevant (Sansosti and Powell-Smith 2006), etc.

In video modelling, one does a video record of target behaviour of a child in a natural setting using a digital camcorder. Subsequently, the video is presented to the child expecting that the child will imitate it thereby hoping that this can lead to promoting socially appropriate behaviour. An exposure to such a video can help a child to memorize and learn to imitate such target behaviour. Also, through video modelling, a child can be offered with a variety of examples that in turn can contribute to generalization (Stokes and Baer 1977). Literature has indicated the potential of video modelling to increase one's ability to use conversational speech (Charlop and Milstein 1989), taking another's perspective into account (LeBlanc et al. 2003), etc. This technique can be a powerful mode of imparting social skills in community and school settings. For example, in community-based settings, video modelling has helped to reduce inappropriate behaviour (Schreibman et al. 2000) in children. Again, in school-based settings, video modelling has been shown to teach one the art of spontaneous social interaction (Maione and Mirenda 2006).

Children with autism often find computer-assisted learning as interesting. Use of computers has been shown to reduce one's inappropriate disposition in a social setting (Whalen et al. 2006) and increase the use of social etiquettes during communication (Bernard-Opitz et al. 2001).

Researchers have shown the effectiveness of computer-based social stories and video modelling (Sansosti and Powell-Smith 2008; Charlop-Christy et al. 2000) to teach social communication skills to children with autism. Once the video was prepared, the researchers (Sansosti and Powell-Smith 2008) presented the social story as self-driven automated PowerPoint slides accompanied with voice over followed by playing of the video. Their results indicate that the computer-based social story and video presentation of target behaviour can improve the social communication skills of participants with autism.

3.3.2.5   Computers for Training in Imitation Skills

Children with autism are often characterized by an inability to imitate. Researchers have pointed out that there is a neural basis of such a disorder with the mirror neurons in the frontal cortex adversely affected (Williams et al. 2001). Such a deficit in imitation is often manifested in terms of lack of behavioural and/or motor-related imitation. Such a deficit can have cascading effects that can subsequently result in difficulties in building social relations, carrying out social interaction and also learning skills in later stages of development (Rogers and Pennington 1991). Again, Carpenter et al. (1998) have reported that imitation can be useful to teach language to children with autism unlike typically developing children and emphasized the importance of addressing imitation deficit at an early age.

3.3.2.5.1   Computers for Imparting Training in Behavioural Imitation Skills

Children with autism have deficit in imitation skills. To address this deficit, conventional techniques using traditional behavioural approaches deliver intervention through discrete trial training. This involves long hours of one-on-one sitting of the child with the therapist in which the therapist sits facing the child while facilitating him or her to exhibit imitative behaviour. This is accompanied with relevant reinforcers.

With the advent of computing technology, researchers have used the computer-assisted platform to administer the imitation skill learning among children with autism. For example, researchers (Vivanti et al. 2014) have used computer to offer a video presentation of an action in which an actor picks up an object kept on a table in front of her. A child was placed in a similar setting with a table in front of him or her and objects (same as that presented in the video) were placed on the table. While the actor picked up an object, the child was expected to imitate the actor and pick up a similar object from the table kept in front of him or her (Fig. 3.11). The researchers recorded the child's behaviour in terms of his or her imitation capability.

3.3.2.5.2   Computers for Teaching Speech Imitation Skill

Children with autism often suffer from inadequate audio-visual integration capability (Williams et al. 2004a, b). By audio-visual, I mean speech (in the form of a continuous stream of sound) combined with gesture and facial expression during a face-to-face social communication. Research has shown that combining auditory speech with visual effect such as that coming from a talking face can be effective in

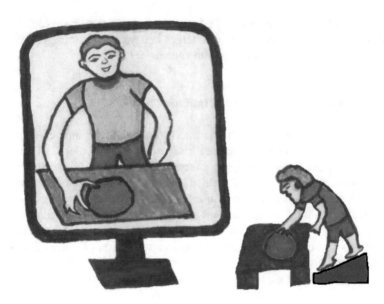

Fig. 3.11 Example of imitating the art of picking up an object from the table

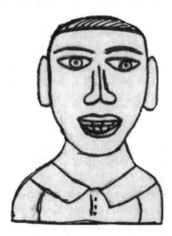

Fig. 3.12 Thematic representation of a computer-generated talking head

offering speech training (Summerfield and McGrath 1984). Again, studies have been carried out combining visible speech with spoken message and this has been referred to as the McGurk effect (McGurk and Mac Donald 1976). It has been shown that perception of speech can be considered as a bimodal process that has a culmination of both sight and sound originating from the speaker (Massaro 1998). In one of the studies by Williams et al. (2004a, b), a computer-generated and animated talking head (Fig. 3.12 shows a thematic representation) empowered with a speech synthesizer was used. The talking head was capable of making precise lip, face, and tongue movements while generating speech. The study was carried out both at home and school-based settings.

3.3.2.6   Computers for Teaching False Belief

The false belief, one of the vital ingredients of Theory of Mind, is critical in the study of a child's development process. Researchers have reported that at a tender age, typically developing (TD) children acquire the ability to attribute belief states to themselves and their social partners (Wimmer and Perner 1983). In contrast, children with autism face milestones with regard to false belief compared with their mental age-matched TD counterpart (Baron-Cohen et al. 1985). Researchers have been pondering whether at least some aspects of the Theory of Mind can be taught to the children with autism so that they can handle various social situations. The passing of the false belief test involves the efficiency with which a child can differentiate between his or her belief (true belief) and belief held by someone else (false belief).

An example of a false belief task can be in which there are two children named Ram and Shyam who are playing with a small toy car. Each of them has a small box. Ram has a blue-coloured box and Shyam has a green-coloured box. While playing with the car, Ram felt like going out to drink water. Before going, he put the toy in his blue-coloured box. In his absence, Shyam wanted to play with the toy and thereby took out the toy from the blue-coloured box. After playing for a while with the toy, he also wanted to go out to have some water. Before leaving, Shyam kept the toy inside his green-coloured box. Soon after Shyam left, Ram came back and wanted to resume playing with the toy car. Now, given this scenario in front of a child named Mahim (say), Mahim is asked, 'Where does Ram search for the toy car?' If Mahim could relate his thoughts properly with Ram's perspective, he needs to say that 'Ram will search for the toy car in the blue-coloured box.' But in reality, the toy car was lying in the green-coloured box.

Researchers have used various experimental studies to administer false belief tasks to children. For example, let us consider a study by Appleton and Reddy (Appleton and Reddy 1996) in which the researchers have exposed a group of children who had failed the false belief tasks to video clips demonstrating such tasks. Also, this was compared with other approaches such as exposing another group of age-matched children (who had failed the false belief task) to reading sessions built around false belief tasks. To administer such tasks, the researchers used 'misleading appearance task' and 'location task'. The 'misleading appearance task was of three types, namely the 'Smarties Task', 'The Egg Box Task', and the 'Milk Bottle Task'. Each container was made to have an object different from the one that an individual can expect. For example, the Smarties tube had a pencil, the Egg Box had a small ball and the Milk Bottle had a toothbrush inside. In this study, the authors first asked the children regarding their thoughts on what was there in each box. This was followed by opening each container and showing the contents inside each container to the child. Again, this was followed by asking the same question to the child. The 'Location Task' was designed to administer the false belief task while changing the location of a target object. Here, the researchers used cartoon representation (in the form of drawings) in which a small girl (Sally) had put some sweets on a table and went outside the room. The other player, John, a small boy took the sweets and kept these in a drawer followed by him leaving the room. Questions were posed to the child by the experimenter regarding the location that Sally can search for the sweets after she returned back to the room. Results of a post-test session indicated that the children exposed to the video clips performed better than the other group. Also, training was able to help in generalizing the task to other scenarios as well.

Researchers have used computers to project false belief tasks. For example, researchers have used Sally-Anne task (Swettenham 1996) to administer the false belief task among children with autism. In this study, Sally had a marble that she kept in a location (A, say) followed by leaving the place. Then Anne moved the marble to a different location (B, say) while Sally was not there. When Sally returned, she was asked regarding the location where she expected her marble to be. In order to pass the false belief task, Sally would be likely to search for her marble by going to the location A (that was false) instead of searching the marble at its actual location. The games were displayed on a computer accompanied with music, text, and animation. A child could interact with the task using a computer mouse. Also, this study offered variations within the false belief tasks. Some of these were the 'False Breakfast Task' and the 'Tom Task'. The 'False Breakfast Task' used a deceptive appearance mechanism similar to the 'Smarties Task'. The task used a cornflakes packet having an orange instead of cornflakes and a milk can having water instead of milk. The 'Tom Task' consisted of four stories. Each story had a character Tom, who had a false belief regarding the type of weather (sunny or rainy) and the time (day or night). A child who was administered this task was expected to estimate Tom's behaviour with regard to the weather and the time. Following the computer-assisted teaching, the children were tested to see whether they have understood the concept behind the false belief task. It was found that the children with autism were able to pass the task in a test scenario in which the training materials were similar to that during training. However, once training materials were changed in the test scenario, the children could not do the task satisfactorily.

Thus, questions still remain on the generalizability of the skills learnt by the child. May be using variations in the display stimulus such as through the use of Virtual Reality might help in the generalization of the learnt skills. Specifically, Virtual Reality can be used to offer variations in 3D computer-mediated simulated worlds that can be realistically rendered. Also, users can interact with these worlds with joystick, mouse, and other external peripherals that can be easily integrated with this platform (Parsons and Mitchell 2002). In fact, Virtual Reality can be used to convey mental states of simulated characters by the use of thought bubbles that have been shown to be promising to help children with autism to pass false belief tasks (Parsons and Mitchell 1999).

3.3.2.7 Computers for Teaching Joint Attention Skill

Deficit in joint attention can adversely affect one's communication skills. For typically developing individuals, joint attention generally develops between 6 and 12 months of age. The term 'joint' refers to the triadic coordination or sharing of information (Leekam and Moore 2001). The term 'attention' refers to the sharing of attention between a child, an adult and an object of interest (Bakeman and Adamson 1984). The triadic exchanges can be both imperative and declarative. Imperative exchange refers to the requesting function, and declarative exchange refers to the awareness in or experience of sharing (Go'mez et al. 1993; Mundy et al. 1993). Children with autism possess milestones as far as both the imperative and declarative exchanges are concerned with the impairment in the declarative type being more prominent (Sigman et al. 1986). Again joint attention refers to the behavioural disposition in terms of response to various cues by social partners such as gaze following and finger pointing (Charman 2003).

Computer-assisted skill learning has invaded the domain of special education for several years (Bernard-Opitz et al. 1990). In fact, computer-based applications have been used from education to learning of establishing eye contact and interpersonal social skills (LaCava et al. 2010; Williams et al. 2002). Researchers have used the computer-assisted medium along with therapist's cuing while administering joint attention skill training (Miller et al. 2018). In this research study, the computer screen displayed the face of a character that started the task by saying 'Look at me' while calling a learner by his or her name. The computer-based system was integrated with an eye tracker that sensed whether the child was looking towards the character or not. In case the child did not look towards the character, then the therapist verbally cued the participant to look towards the character. In spite of the verbal prompt, if the child did not look towards the character, then the therapist used verbal prompt coupled with physical prompting. Finally, the size of the target was increased to cover the entire screen so as to facilitate the child to look towards the cued target. At each stage of this gradually increasing prompt, the therapist offered reinforcement to the child.

Again, researchers have used the computer-assisted collaborative framework to teach joint attention skills while promoting social interaction in children with autism. For example, researchers (Sharma et al. 2016) have used computer-based platform to present visual stimulus such as balloons on the computer screen. The idea was to explore proto-declarative pointing (Goodhart and Baron-Cohen 1993). The pointing gesture of a learner was picked up by an imaging device that was integrated with the computer. To facilitate learning of shared attention (important ingredient of learning joint attention skill), a balloon could be chosen by one of the learners (i.e. a player) (Fig. 3.13 shows the hand position of a player close to one of the balloons) or by two players in the collaborative team. The task required both the players in the team to use their hands to select the same virtual balloon. The aim was to encourage social communication (verbal or non-verbal) between the players. Different reinforcers were offered by the computer-assisted platform. For example, if one player of a team

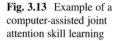
Fig. 3.13 Example of a computer-assisted joint attention skill learning

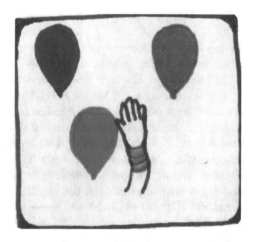

chose a balloon by raising a pointing hand, then a star appeared on the screen. If both the players chose the same virtual balloon, then a multi-coloured rainbow appeared on the screen as a reward.

3.4   Summary

Children with autism are characterized by deficits in social communication marked by disability in various skills, such as imitation, joint attention, etc. Although conventional techniques are powerful, yet, with resource limitation and other factors, getting accessibility to such specialized services might be a challenge for many. Technology-assisted systems can play a complementary role. Investigators are now using technology to develop accessible, quantifiable, intensive, and individualized intervention that is potent to address at least some of the core deficit areas characterizing autism. In this chapter, I have introduced the reader to the technology-assisted systems, namely robot-assisted and computer-based systems that can address various deficits associated with autism. Additionally, I have presented a number of applications of such technology-assisted platforms. Robot-assisted techniques offering 3D embodiment catering to the sense of presence have a myriad of advantages. However, these set-ups are often expensive with difficulty in incorporating variations that might need hardware modifications. Computer-assisted platforms can offer cost-effective interactive medium that can be flexibly programmed to offer individualized services.

Research shows that individuals with autism are often comfortable while interacting with computers since computers can present predictable environment (Colby and Smith 1971; Moor 1998; Powell 1996). Also, computers can help focus one's attention onto the screen while offering a controlled environment in which distractions can be minimized (Murray 1997). Given the fact that many children with autism like to interact with computers and generally prefer to be aloof from social settings, computer-assisted training can be powerful. However, there had been controversy over the use of computers in imparting social skill learning since this might contribute to alienating the children from society (Chen and Bernard-Opitz 1993). But, there is evidence that skills taught through the use of computers at initial stages of skill learning can generalize and translate these learnt skills from the simulated environment to the real world.

One of the ways by which this can be achieved is by bringing in an element of reality in the simulated world. For example, the simulated reality can feature realistic virtual characters and the learner gets to meet these virtual characters and be trained before facing real-life situations. Adding virtual characters that can be flexibly configured to display real-life animations and offered with intelligence using artificial intelligence techniques might enable a designer to present near-to realistic training scenarios in the computer-assisted platform. Such virtual characters embedded in realistic social scenarios can offer a sense of presence to the learner while getting a taste of at least some of the aspects of real-life social settings. This leads the way towards augmenting computer-assisted skill training with Virtual Reality-based platforms. This is because Virtual Reality provides flexibility to the designer to project variations in the skill training environment while controlling the task challenge level for individualized skill training, thereby making training interesting for the learners.

References

Adler J (1968) The study of an autistic child. In: Proceeding of the 3rd annual conference of the American Dance Therapy Association, Madison

Alemia M, Mahboub BN (2016) Exploring social robots as a tool for special education to teach English to Iranian kids with autism. Int J Robot 4(4):30–41

American Psychiatric Association (2000) Diagnostic and statistical manual of mental disorders. American Psychiatric Association, Washington, DC

Appleton M, Reddy V (1996) Teaching three year-olds to pass false belief tests: a conversational approach. Soc Dev 5(3):275–291

Bakeman R, Adamson LB (1984) Coordinating attention to people and objects in mother–infant and peer–infant interaction. Child Dev 55:1278–1289

Baron-Cohen S, Leslie AM, Frith U Cognition (1985) Does the autistic child have a "theory of mind"? Cognition 21(1):37–46

Basil C, Reyes S (2003) Acquisition of literacy skills by children with severe disability. Child Lang Teach Ther 19:27–45

Bekele ET, Lahiri U, Swanson AR, Crittendon JA, Warren ZE, Sarkar N (2013) A step towards developing adaptive robot-mediated intervention architecture (ARIA) for children with Autism. IEEE Trans Neural Syst Rehabil Eng 21(2):289–299

Bernard-Opitz V, Ross K, Tuttas ML (1990) Computer assisted instruction for autistic children. Ann Acad Med 19(5):611–616

Bernard-Opitz V, Sriram N, Sapuan S (1999) Enhancing vocal imitations in children with autism using the IBM speechviewer. Autism 3:131–147

Bernard-Opitz V, Sriram N, Nakhoda-Sapuan S (2001) Enhancing social problem solving in children with autism and normal children through computer-assisted instruction. J Autism Dev Disord 31(4):377–384

Beuscher AV, Cidav Z, Knapp M et al (2014) Costs of autism spectrum disorders in the United Kingdom and the United States. JAMA Pediatr 168(8):721–728

Blocher K, Picard RW (2002) Affective social quest: emotion recognition therapy for autistic children. In: Dautenhahn K, Bond AH, Canamero L, Edmonds B (eds) Socially intelligent agents: creating relationships with computers and robots. Kluwer Academic, Boston, MA

Blow M, Dautenhahn K, Appleby A, Nehaniv CL, Lee D (2006) The art of designing robot faces – dimensions for human-robot interaction. Human robot interaction. Robot Hub, Salt Lake City, UT

Bondy A, Frost L (1994) The picture exchange communication system. Focus Autistic Behav 9:1–19

Breazeal C (2000) Sociable machines: expressive social exchange between humans and robots. Sc. D. dissertation, Department of Electrical Engineering and Computer Science, MIT

Carpenter M, Nagell K, Tomasello M (1998) Social cognition, joint attention and communicative competence from 9 to 15 months of age. Monogr Soc Res Child Dev 63:176

Chandler LK, Lubeck RC, Fowler SA (1992) Generalization and maintenance of pre-school children's social skills: a critical review and analysis. J Appl Behav Anal 25:415–428

Charlop MH, Milstein JP (1989) Teaching autistic children conversational speech using video modeling. J Appl Behav Anal 22(3):275–285

Charlop-Christy MH, Le L, Freeman KA (2000) A comparison of video modelling within vivo modelling for teaching children with autism. J Autism Dev Disord 30(6):537–552

Charlop-Christy MH, Carpenter M, Le L, LeBlanc LA, Kellet K (2002) Using the picture exchange communication system (pecs) with children with autism: assessment of pecs acquisition, speech, social-communicative behavior, and problem behaviour. J Appl Behav Anal 35(3):213–221

Charman T (2003) Why is joint attention a pivotal skill in autism? Philos Trans R Soc Lond B 358:315–324

Chen SA, Bernard-Opitz V (1993) Comparison of personal and computer-assisted instruction for children with autism. Ment Retard 31(6):368–376

Colby K (1973) The rationale of computer based treatment of language difficulties in non-speaking autistic children. J Autism Child Schizophr 3:254–260

Colby K, Smith D (1971) Computers in the treatment of non speaking autistic children. Curr Psychiatr Ther 11:1–17

Costonis M (1978) Therapy in motion. University of Illinois Press, Urbana, IL

Crozier S, Tincani MJ (2005) Using a modified social story to decrease disruptive behavior of a child with autism. Focus Autism Other Dev Disabil 20(3):150–157

Dautenhahn K, Werry I (2004) Towards interactive robots in autism therapy: background, motivation and challenges. Pragmat Cogn 12:12–35. https://doi.org/10.1075/pc.12.1.03dau

Silva P De, Tadano K, Saito A, Lambacher S, Higashi M (2009) Therapeutic-assisted robot for children with autism. In: the 2009 IEEE/RSJ international conference on intelligent robots and systems, Oct. 11–15, 2009, St. Louis, USA

Duquette A, Michaud F, Mercier H (2007) Exploring the use of a Mobile robot as an imitation agent with children with low functioning autism. Auton Robot 24(2):147–157

Eigsti I, Bennetto L, Dadlani M (2007) Beyond pragmatics: morphosyntactic development in autism. J Autism Dev Disord 37:1007–1023

Elksnin LK, Elksnin N (1998) Teaching social skills to students with learning and behaviour problems. Interv Sch Clin 33:131–140

Ferrari E, Robins B, Dautenhahn K (2009) Therapeutic and educational objectives in robot assisted play for children with autism. In: Proc. 18th IEEE Int. Symp. Robot Hum. Interact. Commun. (RO-MAN 2009), Sept. 27–Oct. 2, Toyama, Jpn. IEEE, Piscataway, NJ, pp 108–14

Gabig CS (2010) Phonological awareness and word recognition in reading by children with autism. Commun Disord Q 31(2):67–85

Ganz ML (2007) The lifetime distribution of the incremental societal costs of autism. Arch Pediatr Adolesc Med 161(4):343–349

Gillon GT (2004) Phonological awareness: from research to practice. Guilford, New York

Go'mez JC, Sarria E, Tamarit J (1993) The comparative study of early communication and theories of mind: ontogeny, phylogeny and pathology. In: Baron-Cohen S, Tager-Flusberg H, Cohen D (eds) Understanding other minds: perspectives from autism. Oxford University Press, Oxford, pp 397–426

Goodhart F, Baron-Cohen S (1993) How many ways can the point be made? Evidence from children with and with-out autism. First Lang 13(38):225–233

Goodwin MS (2008) Enhancing and accelerating the pace of autism research and treatment: the promise of developing innovative technology. Focus Autism Other Dev Disabil 23:125–128

Gray CA (1998) Social stories and comic strip conversations with students with Asperger syndrome and high-functioning autism. In: Schopler E, Mesibov GB, Kunce LJ (eds) Asperger syndrome or high-functioning autism? Plenum, New York, pp 167–198

Han J, Jo M, Jones V, Jo JH (2008) Comparative study on the educational use of home robots for children. J Inf Process Syst 4(4):159–168. https://doi.org/10.3745/JIPS.2008.4.4.159

Haritaoglu I, Cozzi A, Koons D, Flickner M, Yacoob Y, Zotkin D, Duriswami R (2001) Attentive toys. International conference on multimedia and expo, 2001

Harris S, Hardleman JS, Alessechrdi M (1990) Teaching youths with autism to offer assistance. J Appl Behav Anal 23:297–305

Heimann M, Nelson KE, Tjus T, Gillberg C (1995) Increasing reading and communication skills in children with autism through an interactive multimedia computer program. J Autism Dev Disord 25:459–480

Heron TE, Okyere BA, Miller AD (1991) A taxonomy of approaches to teach spelling. J Behav Educ 1:117–130

Hetzroni O, Shalem U (2005) From logos to orthographic symbols: a multilevel fading computer program for teaching nonverbal children with autism. Focus Autism Other Dev Disabil 20:201–212

Hodgdon L (1999) Solving behavior problems in autism: improving communication with visual strategies. Quirk Roberts, Troy, MI

Hoffman G, Breazeal C (2004) Robots that work in collaboration with people, to appear in CHI 2004. Workshop on shaping human robot interaction, 2004

Holt S, Yuill N (2017) Tablets for two: how dual tablets can facilitate other-awareness and communication in learning disabled children with autism. Int J Child Comput Interact 11:72–82

Inan FA, Lowther DL, Ross SM, Strahl D (2010) Pattern of classroom activities during students' use of computers: relations between instructional strategies and computer applications. Teach Teach Educ 26:540–546

Ingersoll B (2008) The social role of imitation in autism implications for the treatment of imitation deficits. Infants Young Child 21(2):107–119

Ivey M, Heflin J, Alberto P (2004) The use of social stories to promote independent behaviors in novel events for children with PDD-NOS. Focus Autism Other Dev Disabil 19(3):164–176

Kanda T, Ishiguro H, Ono T, Imai M, Nakatsu R (2002) Development and evaluation of an interactive humanoid robot robovie. In: IEEE international conference on robotics and automation, 2002, pp 1848–1855

Kinney EM, Vedora J, Stromer R (2003) Computer-presented video models to teach generative spelling to a child with an autism Spectrum disorder. J Posit Behav Interv 5(1):22–29

Kozima H, Nakagawa C (2006) Interactive robots as facilitators of children's social development. In: Lazinica A (ed) Mobile robots towards new applications. Pro-Literatur-Verlag, Mammendorf, p 784

Kozima H, Nakagawa C, Yasuda Y (2005) Interactive robots for communication-care: a case-study in autism therapy. In: Proceedings of the IEEE international workshop on robot and human interactive communication, Nashville, Tennessee, pp 341–346

Kozima H, Nakagawa C, Yasuda Y (2007) Children-robot interaction: a pilot study in autism therapy. Prog Brain Res 164:385–400

LaCava PG, Rankin A, Mahlios E, Cook K, Simpson RL (2010) A single case design evaluation of a software and tutor intervention addressing emotion recognition and social interaction in four boys with ASD. Autism 14(3):161–178

Lee S, Noh H, Lee J, Lee K, Lee GG, Sagong S et al (2011) On the effectiveness of robot-assisted language learning. ReCALL 23(1):25–58

Leekam S, Moore C (2001) The development of attention and joint attention in children with autism. In: Burack JA, Charman T, Yirmiya N, Zelazo PR (eds) The development of autism: perspectives from theory and research. Lawrence Erlbaum Associates, Hillsdale, NJ, pp 105–129

Lerman DC et al (2004) A rapid assessment of skills in young children with autism. J Appl Behav Anal 37(1):11

Luyster RJ, Kadlec MB, Carter A, Tager-Flusberg H (2008) Language assessment and development in toddlers with autism spectrum disorders. J Autism Dev Disord 38(8):1426–1438

Magnusson E, Naucle RK (1993) The development of linguistic awareness in language-disordered children. First Lang 13:93–111

Maione L, Mirenda P (2006) Effects of video modeling and video feedback on peer-directed social language skills of a child with autism. J Posit Behav Interv 8(2):106–118

Massaro DW (1998) Perceiving talking faces: from speech perception to a behavioral principle. MIT Press, Cambridge, MA

Massaro D, Bosseler A (2006) Read my lips: the importance of face in a computer-animated tutor for vocabulary learning by children with autism. Autism 10:495–510

McGurk H, Mac Donald J (1976) Hearing lips and seeing voices. Nature 264:746–748

Meltzoff AN, Moore MK (1977) Imitation of facial and manual gestures by human neonates. Science 198:75–78

Miller N, Wyatt J, Casey LB, Smith JB (2018) Using computer-assisted instruction to increase the eye gaze of children with autism. Behav Interv 33:3–12

Miniscalcoa C, Sandberg AD (2010) Basic reading skills in Swedish children with late developing language and with or without autism spectrum disorder or ADHD. Res Dev Disabil 31:1054–1061

Mody M, Belliveau JW (2013) Speech and language impairments in autism: insights from behavior and neuroimaging. N Am J Med Sci 5(3):157–161

Moor D (1998) Computers and people with autism. Communication:20–21

Movellan JR, Eckhardt M, Virnes M, Rodriguez A (2009) Sociable robot improves toddler vocabulary skills. HRI'09, March 11–13, 2009, California, USA

Mueller MM, Olmi DJ, Saunders KJ (2000) Recombinative generalization of within-syllable units in prereading children. J Appl Behav Anal 33(4):515–531

Mundy P, Neal AR (2000) Neural plasticity, joint attention, and a transactional social-orienting model of autism. Int Rev Res Mental Retardat 23:139–168

Mundy P, Newell L (2007) Attention, joint attention, and social cognition. Curr Dir Psychol Sci 16 (5):269–274

Mundy P, Sigman M, Kasari C (1993) The theory of mind and joint attention in autism. In: Baron-Cohen S, Flusberg HT, Cohen D (eds) Understanding other minds: perspectives from autism. Oxford University Press, Oxford, pp 181–203

Murray D (1997) Autism and information technology: therapy with computers. In: Powell S, Jordan R (eds) Autism sand learning: a guide to good practice. David Fulton, London, pp 100–117

Nadel J, Guerini C, Peze A, Rivet C (1999) The evolving nature of imitation as a format of communication. In: Nadel J, Butterworth G (eds) Imitation in infancy. Cambridge University Press, London, pp 209–234

Nikopoulous CK, Keenan M (2004) Effects of video modeling on social initiations by children with autism. J Appl Behav Anal 37:93–96

Norris C, Dattilo J (1999) Evaluating effects of a social story intervention on a young girl with autism. Focus Autism Other Dev Disabil 14:180–186

NRC (2001) Educating children with autism. National Academy Press, Washington, DC

Ogeltree BT, Fischer MA (1995) An innovative language treatment for a child with high-functioning autism. Focus on Autistic Behavior 10:1–10

Parsons CL, La Sorte D (1993) The effect of computers with synthesized speech and no speech on the spontaneous communication of children with autism. Aust J Hum Commun Disord 21:12–31

Parsons S, Mitchell P (1999) What children with autism understand about thoughts and thought bubbles. Autism 3:17–38

Parsons S, Mitchell P (2002) The potential of virtual reality in social skills training for people with autistic spectrum disorders. J Intellect Disabil Res 46(Part 5):430–443

Parsons S, Mitchell P, Leonard A (2004) The use and understanding of virtual environments by adolescents with autistic spectrum disorders. J Autism Dev Disord 34(4):449–466

Payne H (1990) Creative movement and dance in groupwork, vol 18. Winslow Press, Derbyshire, pp 16–17

Ploog OB, Scharf A, Nelson D, Brooks PJ (2013) Use of computer assisted technologies (CAT) to enhance social, communicative, and language development in children with autism spectrum disorders. J Autism Dev Disord 43(2):301–322

Poon KK, Watson LR, Baranek GT, Poe MD (2011) To what extent do joint attention, imitation, and object play behaviors in infancy predict later communication and intellectual functioning in ASD? J Autism Dev Disord:1–11

Powell S (1996) The use of computers in teaching people with autism. Autism on the agenda: papers from a National autistic society conference, London

Preston D, Carter M (2009) A review of the efficacy of the picture exchange communication system intervention. J Autism Dev Disord 39:1471–1486

Quill QA (1997) Instructional considerations for young children with autism: the rationale for visually cued instruction. J Autism Dev Disord 27:696–714

Ramdoss S, Lang R, Mulloy A, Franco J, Reilly MO, Didden R, Lancioni G (2011a) Use of computer-based interventions to teach communication skills to children with autism spectrum disorders: a systematic review. J Behav Educ 20:55–76

Ramdoss S, Mulloy A, Lang R, Reilly MO, Sigafoos J, Lancioni G, Didden R, El Zein F (2011b) Use of computer-based interventions to improve literacy skills in students with autism spectrum disorders: a systematic review. Res Autism Spectr Disord 5:1306–1318

Ramdoss S, Machalicek W, Rispoli M, Mulloy A, Lang R, O'Reilly M (2012) Computer-based interventions to improve social and emotional skills in individuals with autism spectrum disorders: a systematic review. Dev Neurorehabil 15(2):119–135

Robins B, Dickerson P, Stribling P, Dautenhahn K (2004) Robot-mediated joint attention in children with autism: a case study in human robot interaction. Interact Stud 5(2):161–198

Roddy A, Neill CO (2018) The economic costs and its predictors for childhood autism spectrum disorders in Ireland: how is the burden distributed? Autism 5:1–13

Rogers SJ, Pennington BF (1991) A theoretical approach to the deficits in infantile autism. Dev Psychopathol 3:137–162

Sampath H, Indurkhya B, Sivaswamy J (2012) A communication system on smart phones and tablets for non-verbal children with autism. In: Miesenberger K, Karshmer A, Penaz P, Zagler W (eds) Computers helping people with special needs, ICCHP. Springer, Heidelberg, pp 323–330. https://doi.org/10.1007/978-3-642-31534-3_49

Sankardas SA, Rajanahally J (2017) iPad: efficacy of electronic devices to help children with autism spectrum disorder to communicate in the classroom. Support Learn 32(2):144–157

Sansosti FJ, Powell-Smith KA (2006) The effects of social stories on the social behavior of children with Asperger's syndrome. J Posit Behav Interv 8(1):43–57

Sansosti FJ, Powell-Smith KA (2008) Using computer-presented social stories and video models to increase the social communication skills of children with high-functioning autism spectrum disorders. J Posit Behav Interv 10(3):162–178

Scassellati B, Admoni H, Matarić MJ (2012) Robots for use in autism research. Annu Rev Biomed Eng 14:275294

Schreibman L, Whalen C, Stahmer A (2000) The use of video priming to reduce disruptive transition behaviors in children with autism. J Posit Behav Interv 2(1):3–11

Sharma S, Srivastava S, Achary K, Varkey B, Heimonen T, Hakulinen J, Turunen M, Rajput N (2016) Promoting joint attention with computer supported collaboration in children with autism. CSCW'16, February 27–March 2, 2016, San Francisco, CA, USA

Shiomi M., Kanda T, Ishiguro H, and Hagita N (2006) Interactive humanoid robots for a science museum. In M. Goodrich, A.C. Schultz and D J Bruemmer (Eds.), Proceedings of the 1st ACM/IEEE international conference on human-robot interaction (pp. 305–312). New York, NY: Association for Computing Machinery

Sigafoos J, Arthur-Kelly M, Butterfield N (2006) Enhancing everyday communication for children with disabilities. Paul H Brookes, Baltimore, MD

Sigman M, Mundy P, Sherman T, Ungerer J (1986) Social interactions of autistic, mentally retarded and normal children and their caregivers. J Child Psychol Psychiatry 27:647–656

Sigman M, Kasari C, Moore C, Dunham PJ (1995) Joint attention across contexts in normal and autistic children. In: Moore C, Dunham PJ (eds) Joint attention: its origins and role in development. Lawrence Erlbaum Associates, Hillsdale, NJ

Simpson A, Lagone J, Ayers KM (2004) Embedded video and computer based instruction to improve social skills for students with autism. Educ Train Dev Disabil 39:240–252

Stanton CM, Kahn PH Jr, Severson RL, Ruckert JH, Gill BT (2008) Robotic animals might aid in the social development of children with autism. In: Fong T, Dautenhahn K, Scheutz M, Demiris Y (eds) Proceedings of the 3rd ACM/IEEE international conference on human robot interaction. Association for Computing Machinery, New York, NY, pp 97–104

Stokes TF, Baer DM (1977) An implicit technology of generalization. J Appl Behav Anal 10:349–368

Stone WL, Lemanek KL, Fishel PT, Fernandez MC, Altemeier WA (1990) Play and imitation skills in the diagnosis of young children. Pediatrics 86:267–272

Stone W, Ousley O, Littleford C (1997) Motor imitation in young children with autism: what's the object? J Abnorm Child Psychol 25:475–485

Stromer R, Mackay HA, Howell SR, McVay AA, Flusser D (1996) Teaching computer-based spelling to individuals with developmental and hearing disabilities: transfer of stimulus control to writing tasks. J Appl Behav Anal 29:25–42

Summerfield Q, McGrath M (1984) Detection and resolution of audio–visual incompatibility in the perception of vowels. Q J Exp Psychol 36:51–74

Swaggart BL, Gagnon E, Bock SJ, Earles TL, Quinn C, Myles BS et al (1995) Using social stories to teach social and behavioral skills to children with autism. Focus Autistic Behav 10(1):1–16

Swettenham T (1996) Can children with autism be taught to understand false belief using computers. J Child Psychol Psychiatry 37:157–165

Tanaka F, Matsuzoe S (2012) Children teach a care-receiving robot to promote their learning: field experiments in a classroom for vocabulary learning. J Hum Robot Interact 1(1):78–95

Tjus T, Heimann M, Nelson K (1998) Gains in literacy through the use of a specially developed multimedia computer strategy. Autism 2:139–156

Travers JC, Higgins K, Pierce T, Boone R, Miller S, Tandy R (2011) Emergent literacy skills of preschool students with autism: a comparison of teacher-led and computer-assisted instruction. Educ Train Autism Dev Disabil 46(3):326–338

Vacca JS (2007) Autistic children can be taught to read. Int J Spec Educ 22:54–61

Vedora J, Stromer R (2007) Computer-based spelling instruction for students with developmental disabilities. Res Dev Disabil 28:489–505

Vivanti G, Trembath D, Dissanayake CJ (2014) Mechanisms of imitation impairment in autism spectrum disorder. Abnorm Child Psychol 42:1395

Voss C, Washington P, Haber N, Kline A, Daniels J, Fazel A, De T, McCarthy B, Feinstein C, Winograd T, Wall D (2016) Superpower glass: delivering unobtrusive real-time social cues in wearable systems. In: Proceedings of the 2016 ACM international joint conference on pervasive and ubiquitous computing: adjunct (Ubi Comp'16), pp 1218–1226. https://doi.org/10.1145/2968219.2968310

Washington P, Daniels J, Voss C, Feinstein C, Haber N, Winograd T, Tanaka S, Wall D (2016) A wearable social interaction aid for children with autism. CHI 2016, San Jose, CA, USA, pp 2348–2354

Wetherby AM (1986) Ontogeny of communicative functions in autism. J Autism Dev Disord 16 (3):295–316

Whalen C, Liden L, Ingersoll B, Dallaire E, Liden S (2006) Positive behavioral changes associated with the use of computer assisted instruction for young children. J Speech Lang Pathol Appl Behav Anal 1:11–26

Whalen C, Moss D, Ilan A, Vaupel M, Fielding P, Mac Donalk K et al (2010) Efficacy of TeachTown: basics computer-assisted intervention for the intensive comprehensive autism program in Los Angeles Unified School District. Autism 14:179–197

Williams JHG, Whiten A, Suddendorf T, Perrett DI (2001) Imitation, mirror neuron and autism. Neurosci Biobehav Rev 25(4):287–295

Williams C, Wright B, Callaghan G, Coughlan B (2002) Do children with autism learn to read more readily by computer assisted instruction or traditional book methods? A pilot study. Autism 6:71–91

Williams JHG, Massaro DW, Peel NJ, Bosseler A, Suddendorf T (2004a) Visual–auditory integration during speech imitation in autism. Res Dev Disabil 25:559–575

Williams JHG, Whiten A, Singh T (2004b) A systematic review of action imitation in autistic spectrum disorder. J Autism Dev Disord 34(3):285–299

Wimmer H, Perner J (1983) Beliefs about beliefs: representation and constraining function of wrong beliefs in young children's understanding of deception. Cognition 13:103–128. https://doi.org/10.1016/0010-0277(83)90004-5

Chapter 4
Scope of Virtual Reality to Autism Intervention

4.1 Introduction

With increased computing power, modern-day gadgets come with built-in rich graphics that can employ Virtual Reality (VR) to project realistic scenarios to the user. There had been a wide array of VR-based applications ranging from entertainment to intervention, education, rehabilitation, healthcare, etc. Specifically, VR-based applications are no more limited only in the area of expensive toys. Its applicability has transitioned to design of academic modules for education, serious games targeted towards intervention, game engines that can offer varying degrees of challenge to individuals with motor disorders, etc. Since the focus of this book is related to different aspects of autism, in this chapter, I will present VR-based applications targeted towards autism intervention. This chapter also offers a glimpse into the different types of VR-based platforms such as VR presented on a 2D monitor, Augment (Virtual) Reality and Mixed (Virtual) Reality used for training individuals with autism along with their merits and demerits.

4.2 Virtual Reality: Its Use in Intervention

Virtual Reality (VR) has been a widely used candidate for delivery of intervention to individuals with phobias (Parsons and Rizzo 2008) and gaming modules to facilitate understanding of false belief (Swettenham 1996), improve attention (Trepagnier et al. 2006), training on the art of recognizing emotional expressions (Silver and Oakes 2001), social problem solving (Bernard-Opitz et al. 2001), social conventions (Parsons et al. 2005) for children with autism, and many other applications. Researchers have reported that VR can be used to offer ecologically relevant stimuli embedded in different situations for projecting meaningful tasks (Rizzo et al. 2013). In fact, the VR technology is well equipped to design realistic situations that can help

© Springer Nature Switzerland AG 2020
U. Lahiri, *A Computational View of Autism*,
https://doi.org/10.1007/978-3-030-40237-2_4

to trigger real-life experiences while dealing with scenarios of varying degrees of difficulty set in VR-based environment. Here, I present some of the advantages offered by VR making this platform particularly suitable for different applications relevant to children with autism. The VR-based environments offer controllability, reduced sensory stimuli, individualized approach, safety, and a reduction of human interaction during initial skill training (Strickland 1997). Here, I explain each of these terms in the perspective of autism intervention.

4.2.1 Controllability

It is known that children with autism possess sensitivity towards sensory inputs (Dunn and Brown 1997). This might have biochemical underpinnings as found from research studies (Chamberlain and Herman 1990). As far as sensitivity to sensory inputs is concerned, there can be varying thresholds for different individuals. For individuals with lower threshold, a small degree of stimulation can be powerful to trigger the central nervous system to respond. In contrast, for those having higher thresholds, a comparatively larger degree of stimulation can be used to trigger the response from the central nervous system (Corbett et al. 2009). In most of the cases, the children with autism are characterized by high sensitivity towards sensory inputs such as sound, light, touch, etc. This can often hamper their skill learning process. The VR-based environments can be programmed to partially or completely isolate an individual from the normal sensory environment (Rose and Foreman 1999) that can be essential to impart skill training particularly at the initial stages.

Often, individuals with autism are hyper-sensitive to external sensory stimuli such as texture, level of sound, etc. The VR-based environment can be programmed in a way that the level of sensory stimulation can be controlled in an individualized manner so as to suit one's specific needs. Specifically, the audio and video-based information on different aspects related to one's sensory stimulation can be controlled while offering restricted information to the user compared with that in a real-world setting. For example, VR-based environment can control the decibel level of a sound corresponding to an action with the sound being used to draw the child's attention while ensuring that the child is not disturbed on account of hypersensitivity to stronger sounds. Again, as far as the visual presentation is concerned, the VR-based settings can be used to offer visual stimuli in an individualized manner. For example, while teaching a skill to a child with autism, the VR environment can be designed so that the level of distraction in the VR environment is minimized that might be difficult to be achieved in real-life settings. In order to reduce the element of distraction while doing a task that involves interaction with a virtual peer, the VR-based setting can be tuned to control the movement of the agents in the VR world. The agents can appear as 3D humanoid characters or animated versions of inanimate objects that are chosen based on the requirement of the task.

The VR-based platform offers flexibility to a designer to develop training environments where the stimulus can be presented in a controlled manner. Also, the ease of programming can help the designer to develop tasks whose challenge level (that is degree of difficulty) can be controlled so as to suit the task demand. Once, the child has been trained, the VR-based setting can be adjusted to bring in distractions in a calculated manner, thereby bringing the aspects of real world in VR while facilitating in the translation of the skills learnt from the VR world to the real world.

4.2.2   Individualized Approach

Autism is a spectrum disorder in which each child with autism can be unique. The heterogeneity in the disorder can cause one specific treatment or intervention not to be the best for all the children (Stahmer et al. 2011). Also, the variation in the different stages of development of a child might need the intervention strategy to be tuned accordingly. This means that as the child grows, the intervention-related needs might change, and then the techniques used to deliver intervention to the child might need alteration for the intervention to be effective. Thus, researchers have been laying stress on the individualization of intervention that is tailored to the needs of each child with autism (Schreibman and Koegel 2005). The literature review indicates that often, in community-based settings, the interventionist does not use only one intervention approach. Instead, the interventionist can use a combination of evidence-based and non-evidence-based approaches (Stahmer et al. 2005). To individualize the intervention approach, therapists often refer to the information on the pretreatment characteristics related to differential intervention outcomes. In conventional intervention settings, often the therapist tunes her intervention paradigm so as to suit a child's specific need. In other words, the effectiveness of the training depends to a great extent on the individualization in the administration of skill training that can be adapted to one's specific vulnerabilities.

The VR-based training environments can be easily programmed to offer individualized training to promote optimum skill learning. For example, if a child with autism has fear of height that he or she faces while using a lift, the child can be exposed to a VR-based environment to offer skill training to the child on aspects related to riding in a lift. Specifically, the VR environment can be used to project various scenes that one can come across while looking outside the glass walls of a lift moving upwards. While such a setting can help the child overcome the fear in using a lift, it can also help to address issues related to safety, availability of resources, etc. (Parsons and Mitchell 2002). Again, let us consider a child who is afraid of closed spaces. Thus, the VR-based environment can be built to project a small closed room where the child needs to carry out tasks that are interesting to the child. The closed room can have limited windows, low ceiling, etc. While doing the task in that room, the child can realize that the closed space is not causing him any harm and thus can overcome the fear related to closed spaces.

4.2.3   Safety

Ensuring safety of a child with autism while protecting them from accidents and injuries is one of the biggest concerns of parents of these children (Ivey 2004). In certain cases, lack of judgement and atypical sensory interests can cause these children to land up in dangerous situations and be injured (Volkmar and Wiesner 2009). There can be two facets of safety. One can be offering these children with skill learning environments that can be safe for them. The other can be offering them with safety training in daily living skills.

As far as offering safe skill learning environments is concerned, let us consider social situations where the child needs to interact with social peers. It is well known that children with autism face milestones as far as social communication is concerned. Often, in a social setting, they alienate themselves from society since they fear the negative consequences, such as a rebuke from their peers. Specifically, the child is often sensitive to the criticisms from their social partners that in turn might deter their acquisition of the social skills. This in turn can lead to cascading effects in their later stage of development. To explain this social exclusion, let us consider an example in which a child with autism has been asked to play with others in a playground without training the child in skills related to social interaction. In such a case, it might so happen that the child feels out of place and becomes uncomfortable. This can be attributed to the atypical disposition of the child while being amidst other children that in turn can lead to unfavourable repercussions from other children. In such a scenario, the child may become more cocooned within himself or herself that might prevent him or her to mingle with others.

The VR-based training scenario can be useful in such a case. The VR environment can offer a safe skill training platform in which one can afford to make mistakes in the process of learning without facing the negative consequences. Also, VR can be used to project social situations in which the child can be accompanied by virtual humanoid characters (avatars) who can act as social communicators and facilitators. While enacting the role of a social communicator, the avatar can carry out back-and-forth social communication with the child along with giving hints on the basic rules of communication to the child. If the child is successful in communicating his or her thought to the avatar, the facilitator can offer positive reinforcement, such as encouraging statements or clapping, etc. Again, while posing as a facilitator, the avatar can be programmed to point out the mistakes made by the child and encourage the child to practise skill learning without any negative consequences.

As far as safety training is concerned, research indicates that children with autism require direct and explicit instruction on skills related to safety as well as generalizing these skills in real-life situations (Summers et al. 2011). This is necessary since these children face difficulties in learning a skill and also translating the learnt skills from the simulated world to the real world. Researchers have used VR to teach fire safety and road safety skills to children (Kenny et al. 2013). The VR environment can be used to simulate various safety drill situations. For example, in one of the previous studies, the researchers used VR to teach the art of navigation in a building in case of fire (Self et al. 2007). The children were asked to use computer mouse to navigate the building, look out for the exit signs, etc. To see the effect of generalization, after few weeks of training using the VR-based safety drill regime, the children were exposed to a real-life safety drill carried out at their school. Again, researchers have been using VR to teach pedestrian safety, street-crossing in the presence and absence of traffic signal, and following road signs (Saiano et al. 2015). In this study, the VR environment was programmed to display the city roads. A motion capture device was integrated with the VR environment to translate the learner's movement into commands used to control the VR scene.

To summarize, the VR can offer a safe practice environment. Also, the skills learnt can be generalized and translated from the simulated world to real-life situations, such as safe navigation while crossing roads, moving through building in case of fire, etc.

4.2.4   Reduction in Human Interaction

Predictability in one's behaviour has an important role in making effective social exchanges. Predictability refers to the essence of estimating the accurate description of events in the future, and there is evidence from literature that individuals often prefer predictability over unpredictability (Steinhauer 1984). The necessity of adjusting to the complex social relationships and getting knowledge so as to be able to predict the behaviour of social partners are important factors in the evolution of human intelligence. Again, human intelligence enables one to adjust to unnatural social situations since human beings are generally capable of picking up and deciphering cues that can help them in understanding the intentions of other fellow human beings (Dautenhahn 1999).

It is well established that children with autism prefer structure, predictability, and consistency (Iseminger 2009) that is often not the case in reality. Specifically, children with autism often fail to pick up cues and in turn experience lack of predictability while considering the occurrence of events as magical (Sinha et al. 2014). Again, lack of predictability in situations and events occurring in reality often leads to anxiety (Abbott and Badia 1986) that is often the case with children with autism.

If training scenarios have structure, are predictable, and offer consistency, then this can lead to effective skill learning by the children with autism since such a scenario can help them to overcome fear and anxiety experienced by them. Specifically, these children feel comfortable in interacting with robots that can be programmed so that its behavioural disposition can be predictable. Additionally, the robot can offer a 3D embodiment that can lend a sense of presence to the learner. However, such artificially intelligent robots are often very expensive. On the other hand, although interaction with humans offers embodied presence and echoes real-life interaction, humans being natural agents often have unpredictability in their disposition. This unpredictability in the human beings might deter the children with autism from interacting with them. In contrast, the VR environment being controllable can offer preprogrammed tasks for skill learning, thereby presenting a structured and predictable environment to the children (Tartaro and Cassell 2007). Further, the soft bots (humanoid avatars) can be designed to serve as communicators and facilitators, thereby offering a sense of embodiment (Standen and Brown 2005). With the computers now becoming cheaper, VR-based training scenarios have become accessible to the public at large.

4.2.5 Promoting Learning Through Imagery

Children with autism have often been referred to as visual learners (Catherine and Roy 2003). Teachers in special needs school often use visual strategies to teach concepts and ideas to these children. The visuals can be pictures, icons, e.g. black and white cartoon images, photographs, or gestures as a complement to the spoken words so as to help these children to understand the underlying idea (Peeters 1997). The literature indicates that a combination of sight and sound can be beneficial to teach abstract concepts to children with autism (Park and Youderian 1974).

The use of imagery such as visuals, picture cards, etc. has been proven to be powerful tools to promote skill learning in children with autism. This in turn can reduce their need to imagine components (Sherman and Craig 2003; Strickland 1997), thereby contributing to skill learning. This is important since children with autism often possess deficit in imagination. These individuals also prefer pictures over written words (Hodgdon 2000). Again, individuals with autism prefer visual over auditory mode of learning (Cohen 1998). Temple Grandin, author of the book *Thinking in Pictures and Other Reports from My Life With Autism*, stated that pictures proved to be powerful for her for conveying a message.

Visual supports have been reported to help children with autism gain literacy skills (Broun 2004), learn to cook (Orth 2003), encourage positive behaviour (Crozier and Sileo 2005) and signalling to change an activity (Dettmer et al. 2000), etc. Due to the power of using visuals for teaching skills to children with autism, therapists often use picture cards (Fig. 4.1). For example, often, therapists use smiley faces on picture cards to encourage positive behaviour in a child. Again, visuals can be used to communicate that a change in activity in a routine needs to be done. An example of such a visual can be to use a photo of someone opening a tiffin box to communicate to the child with autism that he needs to close the book and take his tiffin since it is tiffin time. Another example of the use of a visual to help a child to plan his task with minimal adult intervention is the use of a work schedule along with Start and Finished folders (Fig. 4.2).

Preparation of the visuals and picture cards can be very tedious. Also, designing these contents with variations might often be challenging. Given the importance of visual presentation during autism intervention coupled with the issues faced in designing the visuals with variations, the use of VR-based systems has become

Fig. 4.1 Use of picture cards

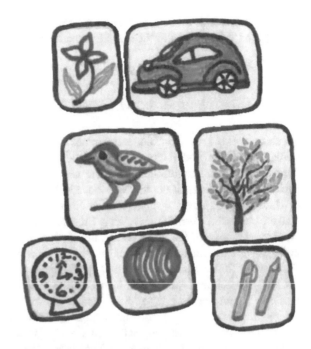

Fig. 4.2 Use of visuals

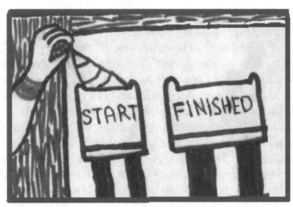

critical since VR offers an avenue to display various objects used for training an individual. In fact, the VR can offer visual and auditory inputs to the user. The VR platform can be easily programmed to present imagery in the form of visuals and soft versions of the picture cards while adding variations to these cards based on the needs. Additionally, VR can be used to project imagery that can mimic real-life environments through realistic rendering. Again, the use of thought bubbles offering a visual presentation of one's inherent thoughts can be effective while administering training in social skills among children with autism (Paynter and Peterson 2013). With the flexibility in design and the versatility in projecting variations within different skill learning settings, this can be potent to foster efficient generalization of skills from the VR world to the real-life situations (Cromby et al. 1996).

4.2.6 Training on Abstract Concepts

An abstract concept refers to one that is not purely physical and is not constrained spatially (Barsalou and Wiemer-Hastings 2005). Understanding an abstract concept might need mental representations. One of the ways to achieve this is through embodied simulations of the abstract concepts (Casasanto 2009).

Understanding such concepts often becomes challenging for children with autism who are characterized with the deficit in imagination (Eycke and Müller 2015) and is considered as one of the important criteria for diagnosis of autism while administering assessment instruments such as Autism Diagnostic Observation Schedule (Lord et al. 2001) and the Autism Diagnostic Interview—Revised (Rutter et al. 2003). Since children with autism have a deficit in imagination, they face problems in mentally transcending time, place, and/or circumstance (Taylor 2013). This is evident from the children with autism being slower than age-matched typically developing children in making acts as part of the pretend play (Jarrold et al. 1996). With a deficit in imagination, these children face issues in learning abstract concepts. In such situations, use of appropriate audio-visual display that can represent the abstract concepts can be useful.

The flexibility in programming offered by the VR platform can be harnessed to bring in programmed variations in the learning scenarios that might be necessary for teaching abstract concepts to these children. This can be applied to teach concepts belonging to different disciplines. For example, let us consider that in a physics class, a teacher is trying to teach concepts on gravitation to an individual with autism. This information being communicated verbally might not be sufficient to teach the concept to the individual. In such a case, VR can be programmed to display scenarios to demonstrate the effect of gravity, such as if there is effect of gravity, an apple (falling from a tree) will move downwards and this can be visually offered using VR. Again, VR can pose questions to the individual by asking 'What happens if there is no effect of gravity?' In turn, VR can be used to display the change in the scenario with no effect of gravity. This is possible, since VR can enable the designer to modify the attributes of objects, add or remove objects programmatically that are invaluable to teach the abstract concepts but might be infeasible in real-world settings.

Another example can be one in which the teacher is trying to teach the laws of electricity to the students. It would be rather difficult for the students to understand the underlying concepts by listening to the instructions offered verbally by the teacher. Instead, the understanding of the concept will be better if visual representation of the phenomenon can be offered in terms of experiments simulated in the VR world along with the observations.

Still, another example can be to add thought bubbles with text. The thought bubbles have been referred to as a mechanism to represent one's mental state (Wellman et al. 2002). Here, the researchers mention that the thought bubbles are a natural and effective way of pictorial representation that can assist a child with autism to understand behaviour and mental states of others. VR can offer a medium in which a virtual agent's thought can be depicted in the form of thought bubbles in simulated social situations so as to hint a child with autism interacting with the agent on what the agent might be thinking. Providing such hints visually would have been difficult in reality (Sherman and Craig 2003).

4.2.7   Complementary Training Platform

It is well established that early intensive intervention can be beneficial for children with autism and their families. This necessitates getting access to specialized intervention services. However, in developing countries like India with a large section of society still living in the rural areas, gaining accessibility to the specialized training centres can be challenging since such centres are available in selected urban pockets. Often the parents need to travel long distances to avail such specialized services. Mostly, the delivery of intervention services involves long hours of one-on-one sitting between the child and the therapist over several sessions that are often expensive and time-consuming. Additionally, one needs to be wary of the deficit related to generalization experienced by these children. To overcome these issues, the child needs to be exposed to various situations in which the skills learnt can be applied. Given such a need, technology can offer a complementary platform that can present varying situations to the child during skill training. The technology can reach even individual households with a promise to address at least some of the core deficits characterizing these children.

The flexibility in Virtual Reality (VR) can enable the designer to design varying educational task environments that can help to address issues with generalization. This can permit delivery of teaching content using audio-visuals that can be entertaining and engaging for the children with autism. Given the restricted availability of adequately trained professionals and difficulty in getting access to scarce special needs schools and training centres, VR can offer a complementary training platform for the children with autism. If VR-based training modules can be developed with valuable inputs from trained professionals, then this platform can be potent to deliver the intervention while using controlled settings. Thus, one therapist can potentially cater to multiple children at the same time with each of them having individual vulnerabilities through the adequate use of VR-enabled devices.

With technological progress and awareness of the use of computers, this digital medium has found its place in many households. Thus, the skill training environments rendered through VR can be implemented in the desktop computers or laptops present at individual households. In such a scenario, the intervention can be carried out, at least partially, by untrained personnel such as caregivers (Standen and Brown

2005), siblings, or peers, thereby ensuring individual households availing the intervention services. This can help to save the valuable time of therapists helping in the intervention. Additionally, this can be used to record the performances of a child during each VR-based task aimed towards training specific skills. In turn, this can help the caregiver to monitor progress made by the child during skill learning using the simulated platform.

4.3   Virtual Reality and Its Augmentation: An Introduction

With advancement in computing power, Virtual Reality (VR)-based platforms have been offered to the users in different forms. This can vary from standalone applications with VR presented on a standard desktop computer or laptop to the more advanced ones in which the VR can be augmented with different kinds of external peripheral devices. These augmented systems can offer a sense of touch added to the visual and audio representation of the context, such as a social scene offering a sense of presence and immersion in the social situation. Examples of different types of VR-based systems are Virtual Reality presented on a 2D screen, immersive Virtual Reality, Augmented Reality, and Mixed Reality among others deployed for a wide variety of applications.

4.3.1   Virtual Reality on a 2D Screen

This refers to the presentation of Virtual Reality (VR)-based object on a 2D monitor of a desktop computer or a laptop. When I mention the word '2D', it might appear to you that the representation of the VR object is similar to a photograph portraying the object from a limited viewing angle. But that is not the case. In fact, the 2D stimulus has in-built depth information of the VR object, thereby retaining the realistic feel in its appearance. In other words, though I refer to 2D, this is actually a 3D virtual object that can be presented on a 2D computer screen while retaining the depth information by displaying its projections with respect to the origin of a 3D virtual world. Additionally, I am not going to present any argument on how the depth information of the 3D virtual object is perceived by the user. Also, VR presented on the 2D screen does not necessarily mean standalone presentations in the form of static PowerPoint display on the computer screen. Here, I am referring to the type of VR platform that can be easily programmed to manipulate different characteristics of the VR objects at any instant based on the study design and interfaced with some of the latest state-of-the-art external peripheral devices. With regard to the programmability, the VR-based environment can be flexibly designed, used to control training environment, offer variety of training modules, etc. to foster effective skill learning. A number of investigators have used such 2D presentation of

VR-based tasks in a variety of applications. Here, I present glimpses of some of these applications.

4.3.1.1 VR Presented on a 2D Screen for Teaching Navigation Skills

Spatial navigation refers to that in which an individual finds out his or her way to move in the environment (Lind et al. 2013). One can use different navigation strategies in daily living, namely route-based and survey-based strategies (Thomdyke and Hayes-Roth 1982). Route-based navigation strategy refers to finding a path based on a learned sequence of landmarks. This refers to the familiar routes, such as finding a way from school to home that one uses almost regularly. On the other hand, the survey-based navigation strategy refers to finding out a way based on mental representations or cognitive maps (Tolman 1948). The route-based navigation can be inflexible and survey-based navigation can be flexible. An example of a survey-based navigation can be finding out a way to navigate in a restaurant environment in which one can find out a way based on cognitive maps. Again, another example can be finding out a way from school to home in which the regularly used route is closed due to maintenance work going on the connecting road. Researchers such as Buckner and Carroll (2007) have argued that navigation can be considered as self-projection that refers to shifting one's perspective to an alternate perspective. However, individuals with autism find difficulty with navigation that has been attributed to the deficit in their ability of doing self-projection (Lind and Williams 2012). Thus, researchers have been designing various computer-based navigation skill training tasks, some of which are set in small covered spaces, some in large open spaces, some in spaces having social gathering, etc.

For example, Prior and Hoffman (1990) offered a computer-based navigation task in a small covered place such as a corridor maze to individuals with autism. In this, the authors have reported that participants with autism faced issues with navigating through the projected scenes. Again, one of the research studies has used large open spaces projected onto the computer screen (Lind et al. 2013). Specifically, here the authors explored the use of survey-based navigation strategy while individuals with autism navigated through a large virtual island using their mental models (Fig. 4.3 offers a thematic representation). The participants were asked to find their way to various target locations marked with specific objects while navigating through the virtual island using a joystick. This task needed one to apply real-world navigation skills where only a part of the world is visible from any particular viewpoint instead of only visual pattern matching to complete the task. In this study, both groups of individuals with autism and typically developing individuals participated. The authors designed two conditions, such as the visible condition and the hidden condition. In the visible condition, the participants were offered some landmarks that they can easily locate and the target object was within their field of view. The participants were expected to remember the location of the target object. This was followed by the hidden condition in which no landmarks were offered to the participants and the participants were expected to find target objects. The

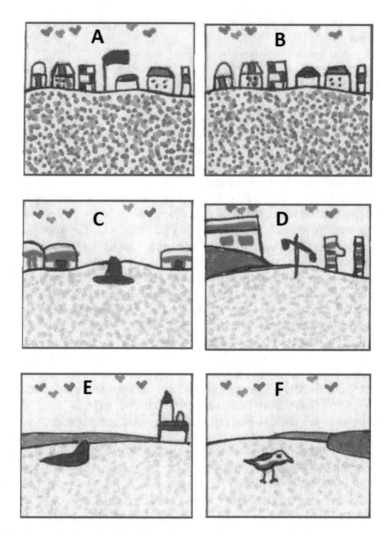

Fig. 4.3 Thematic representation of VR-based navigation task in an open space of a virtual island. (**a, b**) Represent the island in the visible and hidden conditions, respectively; c-f show scenes with target objects under varying conditions

performance in the navigation task was found to be significantly worse for participants with autism than that of their age-matched typically developing counterparts.

Again, one of the applications involved navigation in a closed social space projected on a 2D computer monitor. One needed to follow social conventions while navigating in such a scenario. The idea was to see how individuals with autism navigate in such a scenario. Parsons et al. (2004) used a VR-based restaurant environment projected on a 2D computer monitor for teaching the art of navigation to individuals with autism. Here, the participants were presented a scene from a

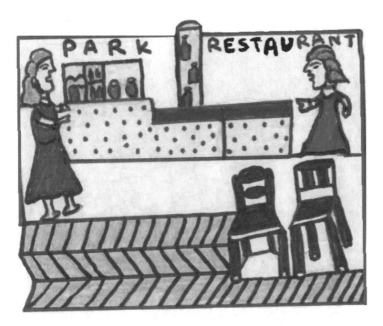

Fig. 4.4 Thematic representation of VR-based training on navigation in a restaurant

virtual café in which there were chairs, tables, menu counter, visitors to the café, etc. The participant was expected to navigate through the café with the help of a joystick, choose a seat, order menu items, take food, etc. using a computer mouse. In this study, the participants were offered with social situations that needed one to adhere to certain social norms such as taking care of one's personal space while moving through the people to go to the menu counter. For example, situations were projected with two people speaking to each other. While navigating in such a situation, one was expected not to walk through the space between the two people, but go en route and utilize the larger open space to the right for navigating to the counter (Fig. 4.4 shows a thematic representation of such a scenario).

4.3.1.2 VR Presented on a 2D Screen for Teaching Pretend Play

Generally, a typically developing child demonstrates an ability to pretend by 2 years of age (Leslie 1987). However, children with autism exhibit reduced spontaneity in pretence compared to their typically developing counterparts (Baron-Cohen 1987). This can be mapped to deficits related to theory of mind in children with autism in which one can be expected to be able to make inferences about another's mind (Perner et al. 1989). Again, there are contrary views in which researchers state that these children do not possess deficits in understanding the pretend play of another individual (Kavanaugh and Harris 1994). However, children with autism fail to show this ability in free play conditions (Jarrold et al. 1996).

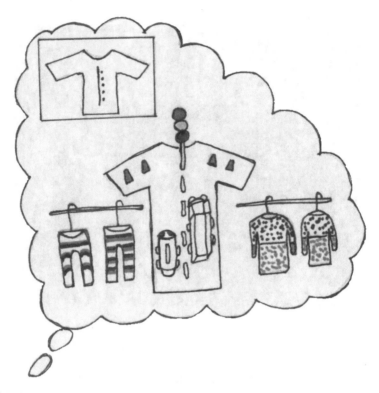

Fig. 4.5 An example of a VR-based scenario for executing pretend play

The deficit in imagination is one of the core limitations characterizing children with autism. Imagination can be defined as a conscious separation of reality from an environment seen with the mind's eye. This can be extended to the art of understanding the symbols and participating in symbolic play. Researcher such as Alan M. Leslie (1987) has proposed three fundamental forms of pretence in real-life situations. These are related to object substitution (i.e. reference), providing false attributes (i.e. truth), and reappearance or disappearance of objects (i.e. existence). The VR-based systems projecting tasks related to pretend play can feature varying combinations or make isolated use of these forms. For example, Herrera et al. (2008) have used VR to project tasks related to pretend play where one of the fundamental forms of pretence, namely false attributes of an object, was used. In this, a play scenario having functional play items (such as an object) and symbolic representation (such as objects that have attributes different from the one in reality) were projected to a child. The 2D VR was used to project a functional object such as a pair of trousers taking the attribute of two arms of a road meeting at a point (symbolic representation). Let us consider another example in which a T-shirt showing a symbolic representation of a three-way junction with a traffic signal and vehicles plying on the road can be used. Figure 4.5 shows such an example. To facilitate this process, one can make use of thought bubbles. The thought bubbles can be considered as a pictorial representation of one's thought. The thought bubbles can assist individuals with autism to understand and find reason for the mental state and behaviour of a social partner (Wellman et al. 2002).

4.3.1.3 VR Presented on a 2D Screen for Teaching Safety Skills

One of the biggest benefits of using VR-based systems is its ability to deliver training content through visual imagery. The VR environment offers a mechanism of presenting visual details organized into a concrete format. This facilitates enhanced visual learning (assisted with imagery) of individuals with autism. Also, VR enables a designer to develop computer-generated environment that resembles scenes from real-life. Thus, VR can be used to teach safety skills to children with autism. For example, researchers have reported that VR-based safety training scenarios presented on a 2D monitor can be effective in teaching safety skills to children with autism (Self et al. 2007). Again, VR-based environment has been used to teach home fire safety (Strickland et al. 2007) and road crossing safety (Strickland et al. 1996) skills.

As reported by Self et al. (2007), two scenarios such as fire and tornado were simulated in the VR environment. Before the safety training, none of the individuals with autism could recognize the visual and auditory cues and react to these cues delivered during a safety drill. In this study, individuals with autism were made to go through training under various conditions. For example, in one condition (Condition 1), the individuals were presented with social stories followed by use of sequenced picture cards and other visuals. With an increase in the training duration, the number of cues such as those given through video, audio, touch, etc. was reduced. Again, in another condition (Condition 2), participants were exposed to VR-based fire and tornado safety scenarios. Similar to that in Condition 1, in Condition 2, with an increased number of exposures, the cues were slowly reduced. This step was followed by a generalization phase in which the children were exposed to safety drills at school. For testing whether the children were successful in learning the safety tips during the previous condition (Condition 1 or Condition 2), the safety administrators used visual cue, such as pointing towards the exit sign, verbal cue, and tactile cue such as touching lightly from behind. The generalization phase was followed by a maintenance phase. In this, the participants were checked to see whether they remember the safety tips 4 weeks after safety training was carried out. Results indicated that both Condition 1 and Condition 2 offered similar outputs. Though both the training strategies were successful, yet the difference between the training environments needs to be considered. In the case of Condition 1, the training was carried out in an environment that was familiar to the participant. However, in Condition 2, the training was delivered in a simulated world. Thus, for those who were exposed to Condition 2, during the generalization and maintenance phases, the training environments were real-life situations that were different from the simulated ones. Also, the training time during Condition 2 (the VR-based modality) was approximately half of that used during Condition 1. In each case, the children could learn safety tips such as moving out of a building in a direction as indicated by safety exits. After offering the training over multiple exposures, the children were able to demonstrate safety skill learning. Thus, VR-based environment could successfully teach the safety skills to the children without being exposed to real-life situations that can be unsafe particularly during the earlier stages of training.

Pedestrian injuries are one of the biggest risks to children in terms of mortality. Pedestrian injuries can be related to inadequate degree of attentiveness, inability to judge the speed of the traffic, prone to risk-taking behaviour, etc. (Sandles 1975; Salvatore 1974). One needs to adhere to traffic rules to commute safely. One of the reports by McComas et al. (2002) has reviewed the use of VR-based environment to teach road-crossing safety skills through visual presentation of such scenarios on a 2D computer monitor. With regard to pedestrian safety, VR can be used to teach children to demonstrate safe street crossing behaviour (Rusch et al. 2002) and tips on using a motorized wheelchair to cross streets (applicable for those with mobility issues) (Inman and Loge 1995) and execute a simple street-crossing-related task (Strickland et al. 1996). Using VR, one can be offered with variations in the street-crossing scenarios. These researchers have designed virtual city with different intersections for teaching different aspects of street crossing. For example, variations were built into the type of signalling used (stop signs, signal lights, etc.), the size of the crossing (single lane, multiple lane), distractions (pedestrians, etc.), etc. Post exposure to such VR-based training scenarios, the participants were immersed in real-life street-crossing situations. The participants were found to learn various aspects of street crossing during the post-training evaluation.

4.3.1.4   VR Presented on a 2D Screen for Overcoming Phobia

Often children with autism have phobias in which these children tend to display avoidance behaviour with regard to the phobic stimulus. To overcome such behaviours, researchers have been using contact desensitization by exposing the child to the phobic stimulus while helping to shape his or her response. Instead of escaping the phobic stimulus, researchers have proposed approach responses coupled with positive reinforcement upon completion of the task (Ricciardi et al. 2006).

VR has shown promise in helping these children to overcome phobias such as agoraphobia (fear of wide, open spaces) and acrophobia (fear of height). For example, VR has been used to project view of a balcony of a two-storey house having a wide open tiled floor and a low fence surrounding it for overcoming agoraphobia (Laky and Lanyi 2003), or a view from a glass elevator for overcoming acrophobia (Laky and Lanyi 2003). Figure 4.6 shows a thematic representation of a VR scene that can be used for agoraphobia, and Fig. 4.7 shows such a scenario for acrophobia. In each of these studies, researchers have reported that most of the children with autism who were exposed to such VR-based training were able to overcome the phobias in real-life situations to a considerable extent.

In many cases, the children with autism might experience specific phobias with loud noise and dogs causing them to become anxious (Joshi et al. 2010; Leyfer et al.

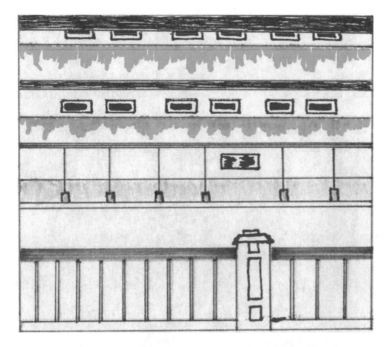

Fig. 4.6 Thematic representation of a VR-based scenario for overcoming agoraphobia

2006; Mattila et al. 2010; Witwer and Lecavalier 2010; Gjevik et al. 2011). Other children might demonstrate phobias related to thunderstorms, vacuum cleaners, and taking a ride in the bus, car, etc. (Mayes et al. 2013). To address a specific phobia such as phobia with a ride in crowded buses, one of the studies presented VR-based situations related to such a ride to participants with autism (Maskey et al. 2014). The VR-based environment was modelled to address the phobia in an individualized manner. Post-test results indicated that the majority of the participants with autism were able to overcome the phobia either completely or to a great extent.

4.3.1.5   VR Presented on a 2D Screen for Social Communication Skill Training

It is known that children with autism are often characterized by deficits in social communication. For example, let us consider situations in which a child with autism is exposed to a park environment. In such a scenario, the child's inappropriate disposition along with failing to adhere to the social norms and etiquettes might cause the child to have an unpleasant experience. Specifically, the child might be bullied by the typically developing children due to the inappropriate reciprocation during social communication. In such a case, the negative consequences might deter the child from participating further in social communication scenarios. Thus, instead

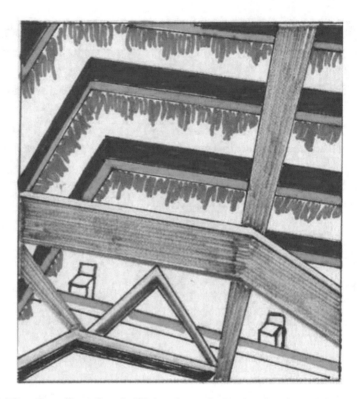

Fig. 4.7 Thematic representation of a VR-based scenario showing view from a lift for addressing acrophobia

of exposing the child to real-life social scenarios, it might be advisable to first train a child in social communication skill away from the real world. In this, the child can be exposed to a simulated world where the child can afford to make mistakes, does not go through the negative consequences, and can explore the world while a facilitator can offer the child with the necessary tips and knowledge on how to interact with peers in such an environment. This can be followed by the child interacting with others in real-world social situations. One of the ways to achieve this is through the use of VR that can offer realistic social scenarios with varying challenge levels to the child. Also, an avatar (a simulated character) can be used to represent the child in the VR environment in which the character can move dynamically inside the VR scene based on the inputs delivered by the child being trained. Also, the avatar can serve as a facilitator to assist the child in the skill learning process.

Researchers (Kuriakose and Lahiri 2017) have designed such scenarios for children with autism. Figure 4.8a shows a snapshot of a VR-based scene that can be used to project real-life social scenarios such as a restaurant environment. The child can trigger the virtual character (the one wearing the blue shirt) to move within the virtual environment by using external peripheral devices. Instead of shouting from a distance, it is desirable that the virtual character (who is a visitor to the

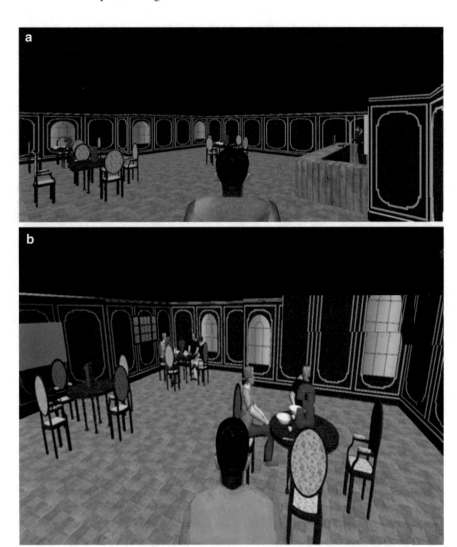

Fig. 4.8 (a) Thematic representation of a VR-based scenario to teach social communication while ordering food. (b) Thematic representation of a VR-based scenario to teach social communication to a child while occupying a seat in the restaurant

restaurant) will walk up to the person standing at the menu counter (the one wearing the black-coloured dress in Fig. 4.8a) to order food.

Subsequently, the VR-based system can be used to project a social scene in which the virtual character (a visitor to the restaurant) walks in an area of the restaurant where most of the tables are occupied. As shown in Fig. 4.8b, the visitor can see three tables numbered as 1, 2, and 3. Of these, Table 1 is totally empty, Table 2 is partially full, and Table 3 is fully occupied. Thus, the child (participant) has few

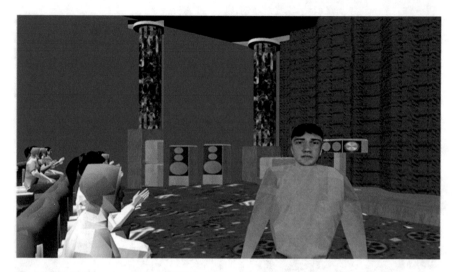

Fig. 4.9 Thematic representation of VR-based scene for teaching social skills while taking a seat at a movie theatre

options. The child can ask the visitor (virtual character with the blue shirt) to sit at Table 1. In this case, a facilitator (system-generated voice) says 'Good choice'. Again, if the participant asks the visitor to sit at Table 2, then the visitor is expected to take permission from the occupants of that table (as a good social gesture), because the other two chairs might be reserved for members who are known to the occupants at the table. In case the child forgets to ask for permission, the child is prompted to take permission from the occupants before occupying a seat at Table 2. This is done by a facilitator who prompts the child to initiate the social conversation by telling the child to ask for permission.

Again, let us consider another social scenario in which a child can be taught how to adhere to social norms while occupying a seat at the movie theatre (Fig. 4.9). Here, the child can trigger the avatar (one with a blue shirt) to move through the seats in the movie theatre. First, there can be a facilitator (system-generated voice) who can say to the child that it is a good time for the audience to enter the movie theatre since the curtain is not yet up and the lights are on. Otherwise, it might cause inconvenience to the audience occupying their seats. While the avatar (one with a blue shirt) tries to take his seat, he might need to move through the seats where people are already sitting. In such a case, the avatar is expected to ask the people sitting on the chairs (who is sitting on his way to his seat) by saying

Hello. Please excuse me. My seat is at the corner.

In case the child does not trigger the avatar to make this request (while following social norms), then a facilitator may prompt the child to do so, thereby training the child in skills related to social communication.

4.3.1.6   Physiology-Sensitive VR-Based Social Communication Skill Training

It is known that children with autism are often characterized by deficits in social communication. The communication-related vulnerabilities can encompass their deficit in making explicit expression of their affective states. By affective state, I mean the feeling of anxiety as an example. By explicit expression, I mean the expression that can be visible through observation. For example, if an individual is upset over something and is anxious, then that might be expressed on his or her face. However, children with autism might not exhibit such an expression. This makes it difficult for the observation-based techniques to decipher the affective state of the child with autism. In such a case, alternate techniques to estimate the affective state of the child might be useful.

Let us consider a child with autism undergoing social communication skill training, and in the process, the child becomes anxious while reciprocating to a social communicator. In such a case, it would be difficult for the child to carry an interaction with the social partner in a lucid manner. Again, such increased anxiety might adversely affect one's learning of social communication skills. Thus, this makes it important to have mechanisms to estimate one's anxiety level while the child is communicating with the social partner. In case of intervention, expert clinicians can use their knowledge acquired from specialized training to estimate the affective state of the child and can modify the intervention paradigm so as to suit the child's need for effective floor-time therapy. However, such estimation is often subjective in nature and depends on the expertise of the clinician to a great extent. One can use alternate technology-assisted tools that can quantitatively estimate the affective state of the child during social communication. One of the possibilities is to use physiological sensing that can offer quantitative estimates of one's implicit anxiety level. Specifically, the autonomic nervous system comprising the sympathetic and parasympathetic branches is activated while an individual is anxious. This in turn can trigger behavioural changes (Kushki et al. 2013) so as to deal with challenging situations with anxiety being characterized by sympathetic activation (Kreibig 2010). The literature review indicates that physiological signals to monitor cardiac activity, skin temperature, electrodermal activity (indicated by sweating), and pupil diameter can be used to offer effective biomarkers of one's anxiety level (Kushki et al. 2015; Raj et al. 2017). This is because, in a state of anxiety, the sympathetic nervous system can have an excitatory effect on one's cardiac function, thereby increasing the function. This in turn can be manifested through an increase in pulse rate. Again, activation of the sympathetic nervous system can lead to vaso-constriction (Kushki et al. 2013) that subsequently affects one's cutaneous micro-circulation causing changes in skin temperature measured from transient variations in one's fingertip temperature. Further, the literature indicates a high correlation between the sympathetic activation and variations in electrodermal effect manifested as perspiration (Kushki et al. 2013) from the skin surface. One's pupil diameter can vary with intensity of light falling on the eyes. However, if the light intensity is kept

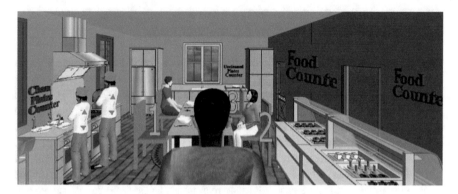

Fig. 4.10 VR-based scenario of a restaurant with buffet counter

constant and an individual is experiencing a state of anxiety, then pupillary dilation might be representative of such a state. Though children with autism might have communication-related vulnerabilities, the physiological signals being involuntary are not affected by the communication vulnerabilities. Thus, physiological signals can offer an undiluted measure of one's affective state. Again, with technological progress, the physiological signals can be acquired non-invasively. Also, the physiological variations, though subtle, can be effectively picked up by the modern data acquisition systems and conveyed to the computer to extract the relevant physiological indices. Subsequently, one can relate the extracted physiological indices to one's affective state in an individualized manner, thereby offering quantitative estimates of the affective states.

If such a tool is interfaced with the VR-based training environment, then the VR-based skill learning can be made sensitive to both the predicted anxiety and the task performance of the child. Mostly, VR has been used to project training scenarios in the standalone mode. Specifically, the VR-based stimulus had not been augmented with modules that can estimate one's affective state, critical for effective social communication skill learning. One of the studies (Kuriakose and Lahiri 2017) has used such a system. As can be seen from Fig. 4.10, children with autism were exposed to various VR-based social scenarios such as a restaurant with a buffet counter, a park environment, etc. The child (participant) could manipulate the position of the avatar (a virtual character with the bluish-green shirt). The buffet counter was at his right side. The avatar would be expected to pick up a clean plate and go to the buffet counter to collect the food items of his choice. Then, he would be expected to go to the seating area and take a seat at one of the tables having four chairs with two of the seats being occupied. While the avatar walked towards the table, the child might feel the need for the avatar to interact with the occupants at the table (as a good social gesture such as asking for permission to sit to make sure that the unoccupied seats are vacant). This might cause the child to be anxious that can be captured by monitoring the child's (participant's) physiology. For example, there might be an increase in the pulse rate, reduction in body temperature, and/or increase

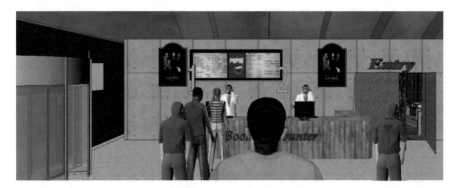

Fig. 4.11 VR-based scenario of a restaurant with menu order counter

in sweating that were measured by a real-time physiological data acquisition system coupled to a VR-based task computer displaying the VR-based tasks. In this case, the VR-based task was made sensitive to the anxiety level of the child. Here, the training environment was made sensitive to one's anxiety that was predicted from peripheral physiological indices extracted from electrodermal (related to sweating), cardiovascular (related to heart rate), and skin temperature. Specifically, when the system sensed that the child was anxious (as estimated from the physiological indices), then the system offered a simple social situation to the child. An example of such a simple situation was one in which tables were totally empty. In this scenario (with reduced challenge), the avatar was only expected to follow table manners, such as proper use of cutlery while eating food without any necessity to interact with others before sitting down at the table. Once the system realized that the child was comfortable, then the VR-based task environment presented the same restaurant with the buffet scene with increased challenge in which the avatar was expected to interact with other members sitting at the dining table.

Again, let us consider another social scenario (Fig. 4.11) in which a child was expected to order the food item from the menu counter and then go to the seating area where waiters served food. Similar to that in the earlier example, a participant (child with autism) could ask the avatar (the one with the blue-coloured shirt) to order the food item. Thus, the VR-based scene displayed the menu counter with two staff members (those with white coats) standing in front of two computers, a queue of people standing to order food, someone having finished ordering and going towards the seating area for having food. On seeing such a social scene, the participant might become anxious and unable to take a decision on what to do. On realizing that the child is becoming anxious (as evident from his physiological indices), the VR-based system triggered one of the staff members (where there is no queue) call the avatar (the one with the blue-coloured shirt) by saying

Hello Sir! How can I help you?

In turn, the participant could ask this avatar to walk towards the menu counter to the right side and order food. In this study, the researchers used one's pulse rate, electrodermal activity, and skin temperature to monitor variation in one's anxiety level while participating in a VR-based social communication task.

In another study, researchers (Raj et al. 2017) used one's eye gaze-related indices to estimate one's anxiety level and in turn made the VR-based environment adapt to the predicted anxiety level. Here, a VR-based environment projected on a 2D computer monitor was interfaced with an eye tracker that can measure one's behavioural looking pattern and eye-related physiology (such as pupil dilation and blink rate). One's behavioural looking pattern can be quantified in terms of the fixation duration towards different regions of interest of the presented visual stimulus. This is because one's fixation towards the face region of a social communicator has been reported to cause anxiety (Garner et al. 2006) among individuals with autism. There is evidence from the literature which shows that individuals with autism exhibit reduced fixation towards salient social cues while carrying out communication with their social partners (Norbury et al. 2009). Again, eye-related physiological indices, such as pupil diameter and blink rate, have been reported to be autonomic measures of one's anxiety (Tsai et al. 2007). Here the researchers have exposed participants with autism to VR-based social scenes such as a birthday party in which an avatar (representing the participant) goes with birthday gift and hands it over to the birthday boy. On entering the room decorated with balloons, cakes, and many guests, the participant might become anxious. This can be sensed by the VR-based system by monitoring the participant's gaze fixation pattern, pupillary dilation, and blink rate. In turn, the system can trigger the birthday boy to walk towards the avatar (representing the participant) and say to him

Welcome to the party. It is really nice to see you here.

Also the VR-based system can adaptively offer tasks of varying challenges to the participant, thereby helping the participant to learn social communication skill while ensuring that the participant is not anxious and is comfortable. This is necessary to facilitate effective skill learning.

The researchers have reported positive contributions of physiology-sensitive VR-based systems in terms of social communication skill learning among the participants with autism. Results of a post-survey (after 2 months of the VR-based skill training) administered by asking the caregivers of these children (who were exposed to the VR-based social communication skill training) indicated that the children with autism showed improvement in such skills in real-life settings (Kuriakose and Lahiri 2017).

With the cost of computers going down without compensating the computing power, graphics, etc., use of VR-based training environments presented on a 2D screen has become affordable. Again, with the cost of computers going down, the increase in competence in the use of computers, and introduction of computing in the school level curriculum, now many hospitals and special needs schools have computing facilities. This has enabled clinicians to offer VR-based training environment to the users at schools, hospitals, and even at an individual household level.

Additionally, increased technological progress has enabled the VR environments displayed on desktop monitors to be coupled with cost-effective computer peripherals. Thus, instead of VR environments controlling virtual objects, thereby allowing users to serve as audience with minimal control on the VR environments, the integration with peripheral devices is empowering the users with a capacity to control the VR environment. Specifically, the user can be an actor who can change the VR environment. In turn, the VR environment is becoming truly interactive from the user's perspective. In other words, this lends a feeling of immersion to the user in the VR environment. Proponents of immersive technology often argue about the extent of immersion or the sense of presence while interacting with the VR world projected on a computer screen. Research has indicated a number of applications of immersive VR in the areas of entertainment, education, etc. for children with autism.

4.3.2 Immersive Virtual Reality (Immersive VR)

Immersive VR gives the user a feeling of being a part of the VR world. Immersive VR can be delivered to the user by different modalities such as Head Mounted Display (HMD), Cave Automatic Virtual Environment (CAVE), etc. A number of investigators have used HMDs for teaching skills to neurotypical individuals (Colzato et al. 2010; Bergeron 2006; Ai-Lim Lee et al. 2010). The Cave Automatic Virtual Environment (CAVE) is another example of immersive VR. Unlike the HMD, the CAVE presents stereoscopic pictures of an environment on the walls of a room. This permits the user to interact with the virtual environment while enjoying a sense of immersion (Vafadar 2013).

There have been reports pointing to the issues such as Cybersickness associated with immersive VR (Pot-Kolder et al. 2018). The tracking position and orientation of the user using the peripheral device need to be communicated to the VR world. Any delay in this rendering in the VR scene will appear as substantial lag, thereby affecting the tracking accuracy and causing flicker (LaViola 2000). This can be attributed to the issues related to seamless integration of peripheral devices with the VR world. Consequently, this might lead to unpleasant symptoms such as headache, nausea, vomiting, etc. of varying intensity and duration (Rebenitsch and Owen 2016). However, with the latest developments in the immersive technology, most of these deficits have been addressed to a considerable extent. Thus, this is now being used in specialized applications for training purposes.

4.3.2.1 Immersive VR for Teaching Shopping Skills

The shopping skill can be considered as a community skill. Training in the shopping skills can be offered in controlled non-community-based settings or in community-based settings. Teaching of shopping skills in community-based settings can include modules on reading aisle signs and finding out the items of the grocery as required by the shopper, checking out at the payment counter, and making the necessary payment for the groceries or other items purchased, etc. When children with autism

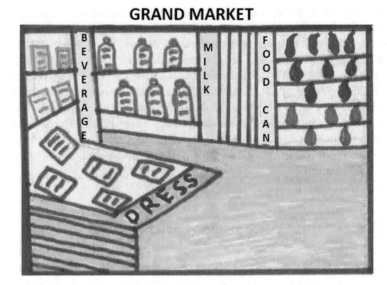

Fig. 4.12 Thematic representation of a VR-based shopping scenario projected using immersive VR

are exposed to supermarket scenarios, they face difficulties with planning their pocket money, finding out and selecting the products of choice, commuting between the aisles having other buyers while experiencing discomfort.

Although it is always beneficial to teach shopping skills in real-life community shopping centres, yet the behavioural repercussions of these children might be so intense that it is preferable to first teach them such skills in a simulated environment. One of the ways to achieve this is to teach them shopping skills by immersing them in realistic VR environment. The aim of the immersive VR-based training will be to facilitate them in learning the skills to safely do shopping. One such example is a study by Adjorlu et al. (2017) in which individuals with autism were exposed to a supermarket scenario projected onto Head-Mounted Display (HMD) glasses. The HMD is a device that fits onto one's head and presents stereoscopic video to each eye of a user, thereby providing a sense of being immersed in the VR scenario. Immersive VR is offered by augmenting VR-based graphical user interface with the HMD. Figure 4.12 shows a thematic representation of such a scenario.

4.3.2.2   Immersive VR for Exergaming

Physical exercise has been shown to be powerful in contributing to improved executive functioning in neurotypical individuals (Hillman et al. 2004). Also, physical exercise has been shown to reduce repetitive behaviours in individuals with autism (Lang et al. 2010). With increased use of electronic media, children spend a lot of time sitting with the electronic gadgets, thereby decreasing their physical activity. Again, most of the children with autism prefer to be sedentary. In fact, research studies have reported that these children show much less physical activity during recess hours as compared to typically developing children (Pan 2008). Also, studies have shown that the children with autism participate in very limited parent-reported physical activities than that of the typically developing children (Bandini et al. 2012). Reduced physical activity coupled with a sedentary lifestyle can be associated with both short-term and long-term health consequences (Jones et al. 2017). The health consequences can be in terms of cardio-metabolic risk, reduction in psychosocial well-being, poor cognitive functioning, poor weight status, etc. (Hinkley et al. 2014). The literature review indicates that exergaming can lead to an improvement in mental health by reducing anxiety and depression for individuals with autism (Mazzone et al. 2013).

Offering these children with facilities of exergaming in which one can do physical exercise that is entertaining is important. This can motivate these children to be non-sedentary. One of the research studies have used immersive VR to expose the children to a scenario in which objects (such as satellites) appeared moving towards them (Finkelstein et al. 2010). This uses a Cave Automatic Virtual Environment (CAVE) technology having stereoscopic projectors, polarized glasses, etc. A CAVE is a small space having at least three walls that can act as big monitors. Unlike the HMDs, the CAVE offers a user with a wide field of view and the users can have the flexibility to move around in the space, thereby having naturalistic experience. In the study by Finkelstein et al. (2010), the researchers projected scenes from space in which one can have the experience of planets, asteroids, stars, etc. that are speeding towards the child. The task needed the child to jump over, move under, or avoid the virtual object speeding towards him or her while scoring points in the game. In this, the child was expected to move and change his or her location so as to avoid collision with the objects moving towards him or her (Fig. 4.13 shows a thematic representation). A collision with the speeding object would infer that the child was not appropriately dodging the virtual object racing towards him or her. In such a case, the task platform penalized the child by reducing the performance score. The game was designed with variations. In certain cases, purposeful collision was required to score points. For example, one needed to do certain actions in order to shoot laser beams towards speeding objects. The actions could be moving the arms back and forth, jump, raise arm, pump, etc.

In another study, researchers have used Head Mounted Display integrated with Virtual Reality and these were coupled with a 3D natural trampoline (Tiator et al. 2018). It recorded one's jumping height. This study reported that such a system can offer a safe and interesting jumping experience without any simulator sickness.

4.3.2.3   Immersive VR for Teaching Navigation Skill

Everyday, we navigate for different purposes, such as navigating to the workplace by road, navigate buildings for going to the classroom, navigate buildings or spaces for safety (say in the case of an outbreak of fire), etc. Thus, navigation is part and parcel

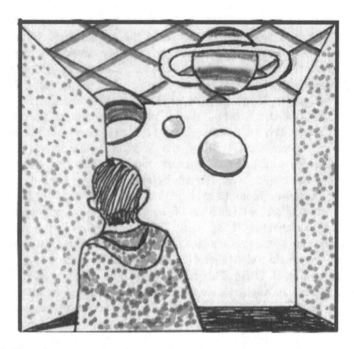

Fig. 4.13 Thematic representation of exergaming projected in immersive VR

of our daily commute. While 2D VR (that presented on a desktop monitor) can be used to teach navigation skills (as discussed in this chapter earlier), immersive VR also finds its place in addressing such skill deficits of individuals with autism. In fact, immersive VR can offer one with real-life experiences that might not be possible in the strictest sense with the non-immersive VR. Specifically, one can roam about freely and explore the environment projected by the immersive VR-based world.

In one of the studies, a Cave Automatic Virtual Environment (CAVE) offering immersive reality was used to teach children with autism the art of navigating through traffic while crossing a busy road (Matsentidou and Poullis 2014). Figure 4.14 shows a thematic representation of such a VR-based scene. This environment was presented to individuals using CAVE iCube, 3D glasses, and an Xbox controller. When the user moved through the environment, the information was communicated to the system that in turn changed its projected scene in front of the participant. Due to the 3D glasses, the user could witness a 3D view of the world presented to him or her. In this, a child was taught the steps required in crossing a busy street with cars and other vehicles plying on it. The steps were to look for the signal and wait for the traffic to stop before crossing the road. When the traffic stopped, the child was taught how to interpret the signal lights and then cross the street. In one scenario, the child was assisted by an educator. Once the child gained knowledge on the traffic rules and used that knowledge for crossing the street, immersive VR presented a situation to the child in which the child was expected to safely cross the street on his or her own. In this way, immersive VR was used to

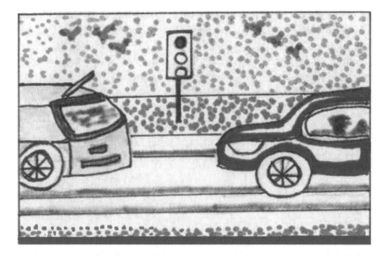

Fig. 4.14 Thematic representation of VR-based training for navigation to cross a street

expose the child to real-life scenarios with an aim to facilitate the child to learn various skills necessary for daily living.

4.3.2.4 Immersive VR for Teaching Locomotion

While individuals with autism are exposed to various navigation-related environments, it is also important to study the modality of locomotion that can be useful for these children while exploring the virtual world. Thus, Bozgeyikli et al. (2016) have investigated the topic of locomotion in the VR environment by immersing participants with autism to different modalities of locomotion within an immersive VR environment. Specifically, these researchers explored eight different locomotion modalities, such as (1) Redirected Walking: This refers to the discrepancy in the dimension of the VR space and the tracked physical space. This can be achieved by manipulating the view projected to the user so that the user physically remains within the limits of the physical tracked area. (2) Walk-in-Place: This refers to gesture of walking without moving forward or backward. The direction of locomotion is generally decided from the direction of walk, or head or the torso of the user. (3) Joystick: This refers to the low-cost alternative to simulate locomotion. Displacing the Joystick handle in different directions can result in the locomotion of the user in the simulated world. (4) Stepper Machine: This was a device that one can stand on and use to step forward. The movement of the stepper machine was picked up by an optically coupled arrangement. The direction of locomotion depended on the direction of head, and turns were simulated by the user by turning his or her head through limited angles. (5) Point and Teleport: This needed one to simply use a pointed gesture using the arm and finger. The locomotion was triggered by using a controller that sensed the user's gesture. (6) Flying: This refers to the hand gesture, such as triggering locomotion by raising one's arm till the shoulder height. (7) Hand Flapping: This refers to the hand flapping that is commonly exhibited by children with autism. The flapping can be done at any height of the body, such as at shoulder height, at the hip height, etc. Any flapping of the user's hand will be read by the controller to trigger locomotion in the VR environment. (8) Trackball: This refers to the use of trackball devices for triggering locomotion in the VR world. A study carried out with individuals with autism revealed that they liked the 'Joystick' and 'Point and Teleport' the best. This was followed by them liking the 'Walk-in-Place' and 'Trackball'. However, they were not in favour of using the 'Flying' and 'Hand Flapping' gestures for triggering locomotion in the immersive VR environment.

4.3.2.5 Immersive VR for Teaching Social Communication Skills

As mentioned earlier, children with autism are often characterized with deficit in social communication skills. Investigators have been exploring the use of immersive VR to offer social communication skill training to children with autism. For example, in one of the studies, the researchers (Halabi et al. 2017) have used immersive VR to teach various social skills related to classroom communication to children with autism. Here, the authors have used various types of immersive VR such as Head Mounted Display that comes with the Oculus Rift and the CAVE Immersive display. The participants were asked to participate in role-play, turn-taking, and reciprocation during social communication. This took a child through different steps in a communication process such as going inside a school building, entering a classroom, and meeting a teacher (avatar) who greeted students (avatars) in the virtual classroom to which the students respond back either verbally or through animation. After presenting such a training scenario to the child, the teacher (avatar) greeted the child by calling his or her name and waited for the child to respond back. The child's response was picked up by using video and/or audio techniques that were integrated with the immersive VR environment. Figure 4.15 shows a thematic representation of such a VR-based communication. Results indicated that the participants with autism were in favour of the CAVE environment that was much less intrusive than the HMD for the participant. Specifically, as far as the feeling of immersion was concerned, the CAVE environment topped the list with the response time (from the participants while interacting with the environments) being least inferring faster response in comparison to that with the HMD.

4.3.2.6 Immersive VR for Imparting Subject-Specific Education

We know that children with autism are visual learners. Thus, certain topics that might be abstract in nature might be difficult for the children to understand without visual imagery. Immersive VR can be used to offer education in specific academic

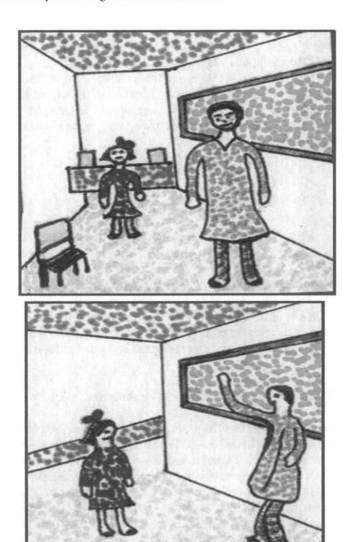

Fig. 4.15 Thematic representation of immersive VR-based training for social communication in a classroom setting

subjects by offering visualization of abstract concepts. This can be valuable for both children with autism and typically developing children. One of the research studies (Pirker et al. 2013) has presented a learner-centric immersive VR environment to offer education in topics and concepts from physics. The researchers used open source Open Wonderland (http://openwonderland.org). The authors present an example of a topic from physics such as Faraday's Laws being taught to the students using immersive VR. First, the students met in small groups and initiated the learning process while going through an acquisition of basic knowledge and improvement in the conceptual understanding, followed by monitoring the progress in the learning of the students. For giving the basic knowledge, first, the system offered videos and documents on the basic concepts. To acquire an improved understanding of the concepts, participants were allowed to take part in simulated experiments. For the purpose of assessment, the system presented questions (on the concepts taught) to the students.

4.3.3 Augmented Reality (AR)

Like immersive VR, Augmented Reality (AR) changes one's perception about the environment. However, unlike immersive VR, the perception about the user's presence is preserved. In other words, unlike immersive VR, AR does not translate the user to a different situation (that is projected to the user). The AR mixes aspects of reality with that of the simulated world, thereby reducing the information content compared to that of immersive VR, which in turn makes AR more suitable for children with autism (Herrera et al. 2006). A number of researchers have been investigating the applicability of AR for skill learning by individuals with autism.

4.3.3.1 AR for Teaching Self-Awareness, Postures and Imitation

Self-awareness can be considered as a concept of self. Children with autism lack in the awareness of the psychological self (Williams 2010). In some cases, children with autism are found to have reduced awareness of their own intentions, and this has been found to be directly related to their deficit in understanding the mental state of a social partner. Again, the ability to imitate is adversely affected in children with autism. Specifically, children with autism face difficulties in imitating actions of others. This has been attributed to their impaired understanding of the organization of movements, thereby resulting in an abnormal representation of actions (Smith and Bryson 1994). One's intact ability to imitate is important since this can be considered as a precursor of achieving developmental milestones, such as symbolic thought and language (Piaget 1952).

Given these deficits, investigators have been using AR to address these skill deficits. For example, in one of the studies, Casas et al. (2012) have used AR while integrating motion capture device called Kinect (comprising of cameras that can provide position and depth information) with a computer-based environment to teach self-awareness, postures, and imitation to individuals with autism. The idea was to help the children to learn their own body schema. To make the skill training task interesting, the researchers designed few playful activities involving body postures and imitation. Using the motion capture camera, one's body movements were communicated to a virtual avatar, which in turn reflected one's movements

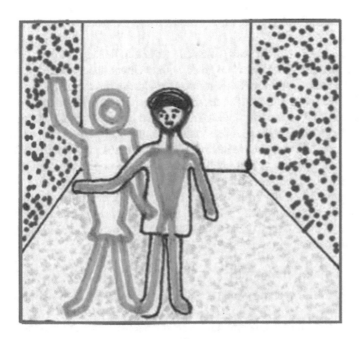

Fig. 4.16 Thematic representation of AR-based training for posture

done in the physical world. This system could portray two users, such as the child and the teacher. While teaching body postures, the task given to the user was to make a posture so as to match with that as demonstrated by the teacher (depicted on the screen). In this, the user was expected to follow the posture of an avatar displayed on the computer screen by imitating the posture. In some cases, the avatar can be in the form of a shadow that guided the user to correctly imitate the posture. Figure 4.16 shows a thematic representation.

4.3.3.2 AR for Teaching Pretend Play Skills

Pretend play can be considered as a meta-representation related to the cognitive basis of the development of the theory of mind in a child (Leslie 1987). Children with autism face milestones in the pretend play skills. Of course, there are debates on whether this deficit can be observed in prompted and unprompted situations. Generally, the spontaneity with which children with autism use toys as agents or substitute one object with the other is considerably different from that exhibited by typically developing children (Rutherford and Rogers 2003). Specifically, children with autism often do not use toys, such as a doll as an agent.

Researchers have used AR to teach pretend play skills to individuals with autism (Bai et al. 2015). A marker-based video camera running at 30 frames per second was used to implement this study. The idea was to overlay an image of an object, such as a train, a car, an airplane, etc. on a piece of wood that was manipulated by a child participating in a task.

In this, a play situation was projected to the individual in which a play object, such as a wooden block, was projected with a virtual alternative (e.g. a car). The child interacting with the AR environment could use the alternative to manipulate the digital scenarios. Using video techniques, the AR was programmed to project an alternative virtual view of the object. Thus, a child could participate in a pretend play situation by moving a vehicle for a rescue operation (say). The object was a block of wood that the child could move into reality (say on a table top) and the AR projected it as an airplane in the virtual environment. Also, to add to the reality of the AR environment, the researchers programmed the propellers and the tyres of the airplane to be dynamic when the child began moving the wooden block on the table top. Thus, in one case, the researchers projected a rescue operation scene in which the user was expected to participate in the pretend play by moving the airplane in the virtual environment to rescue the people trapped in the fire.

4.3.3.3   AR for Teaching Non-verbal Social Communication Aspects

When we refer to the social communication related to recognizing emotional expression, two things come to our mind. Specifically, these are the verbal and non-verbal aspects. By verbal, I mean that the emotional feeling that is communicated verbally. For example, if someone is feeling happy, then the individual can express that verbally by saying

I feel happy today

Sometimes, the mode of expression can be non-verbal. Let us take the same example. Thus, if one feels happy, then that individual can express his emotion by demonstrating a smiling face. Children with autism face milestones in decoding the non-verbal aspects of communication during social interaction. This can be partially attributed to their atypical looking pattern in which they have a tendency to avoid the social stimuli, such as the face of the social partner showing an emotional expression. Another form of non-verbal communication can be the view of a social situation with which an emotion can be associated. For example, the view of someone looking down aimlessly in a park might indicate that the individual is thinking something or is in a pensive mood. Still another form of non-verbal communication can be the use of body movements. For example, the view of someone fighting with another person might convey that there is a feeling of anger that in turn has resulted in a fight.

Researchers have coupled AR with video modelling to teach non-verbal social communication aspects such as decoding facial emotional expression, emotions inherent in social situations, and those represented by body movements to individuals with autism (Chen et al. 2016). Here the researchers have used markerless natural tracking. In this, the users are exposed to a story book containing photos of clippings of a video. The child (user) can read the story book and then can hold an

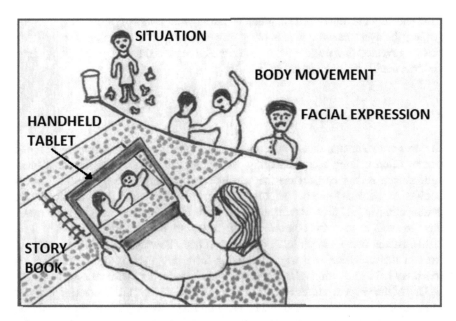

Fig. 4.17 Thematic representation of AR-based stimulus for teaching non-verbal aspects of social communication

Android-based tablet device on the story book. This will cause the tablet displays the realistic scenario in AR (Fig. 4.17) through video modelling and this had been reported to be very engaging for a child.

Through the AR interface, the system offered an extended view of the social aspects of the story and also helped the users to focus on the vital aspects of the videos by restricting the user's attention.

4.3.3.4 AR for Teaching Daily Living Skills

Often, children with autism face difficulties in carrying out their activities of daily living, such as brushing of teeth, causing them to be dependent on the caregiver in daily lives. Given the fact that these children are good visual learners, AR can be used to teach these children some of the activities of daily living through the use of imagery. Thus, the children can learn the tasks both by seeing and doing the tasks.

For example, AR can be used to teach brushing of teeth to the children with autism. Researchers (Cihak et al. 2016) have used an iPod-based AR application to demonstrate the steps that one need to follow to carry out brushing of teeth on one's own. Here, marker-based AR coupled with video clips was used. In this, the steps were presented pictorially beside a sink where the child was expected to carry out the brushing action. The AR application offered a live video representation that the child can follow to learn the art of brushing his or her teeth. The video showed a view of a child enacting the role of brushing her teeth following the steps of brushing, thereby guiding the user (the child who is being trained) in the art of brushing. A post-study session revealed that even 9 weeks after the AR-based training on brushing teeth, children could retain the learnt skill.

4.3.3.5   AR for Exergaming

Children with autism prefer to spend long hours interacting with computers or video games, often making them sedentary. Sometimes, it is not necessarily that these children are sedentary because they do not like to be physically active. This is because of the social and behavioural impairments that restrict these children from participating in physical playful activities with other children that in turn causes them to sit in front of the computers, television, etc. for long duration (Must et al. 2013). Again, parents of children often report that allowing these children to sit in front of the television is a way of calming them down (Nally et al. 2000). Such sedentary habits are often related to their Body Mass Index (BMI) scores.

One of the ways to address this is to develop modules that are interesting in terms of visual inputs and can offer one with an opportunity to carry out physical activity. Thus, researchers have come up with the concept of VR exergaming. This can be delivered by using different techniques, such as the CAVE, Kinect sensor, the Wii-based technology, etc. The CAVE technology as mentioned earlier in this chapter (while discussing application of immersive VR in exergaming) though powerful is often very expensive, has set-up limitations, etc. Another alternative in developing such exergaming platforms can be the use of imaging techniques, such as Kinect that can track one's movement in the physical space.

4.3.3.5.1   Kinect-Assisted AR for Exergaming

The Kinect device can convey movement-related information of a user to the VR-based environment, thereby offering a sense of immersion to the user. This can be an interesting way to include physical activity in the VR-based task environment (Sandlund et al. 2009). The tasks are designed as motion interactive games in which individuals with a sensorimotor deficit need to move their body in order to interact with the game environment. The overall idea is to promote physical activity in the users. For example, researchers have come up with exergames named as SensoryPaint and FroggyBobby (Tentori et al. 2015). The SensoryPaint showed a mirror projection of the user on the wall. The colour of the reflection changed to indicate the variation in the distance of the user from the wall. Users could use balls as paintbrushes having different sizes, textures, and colours to make drawings either using free form or while following certain templates. The SensoryPaint used Kinect sensor and computer vision techniques. This used the depth camera of the Kinect sensor to identify whether the ball carried by the user had hit the wall and to project the user's shadow on the wall. Added to the visual output, this exergaming

a **b**

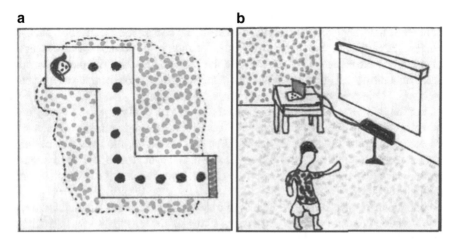

Fig. 4.18 Thematic representation of (**a**) Kinect-assisted exergaming and (**b**) Kinect-based setup

environment played sounds so as to make the task interesting. The task performance was evaluated in terms of performance scores. The FroggyBobby needed a child to move his or her arms in a coordinated fashion, thereby triggering an avatar's (here a frog) tongue to catch flies. Various levels of task challenge and prompting were part of the task design. Using the Kinect SDK, the researchers computed all the joint positions of the user's arm in 3D space while the user participated in the task. Both these exergames were designed to motivate the users to make fine motor and gross motor movements while playing the games.

Again, investigators such as Altanis et al. (2013) designed a Kinect-based gaming environment for children with learning disabilities. Here, a child was expected to undertake horizontal, vertical, and diagonal movements to drive a girl along predefined paths as displayed on the visual stimulus (Fig. 4.18a). The red dots shown along the centre of the path were to help a child avoid colliding with the boundaries of the path. The therapist was given the freedom to choose the type of path (i.e. horizontal, vertical, and diagonal), the time duration for task completion, the width of the path, and the length of the path to be traversed by the child. Thus, various task challenge levels could be manipulated by the therapist based on the training need. The basic set-up consisted of using a Kinect sensor placed on a stand kept on the floor and connected to a computer that in turn was connected to a TV or a projector screen (Fig. 4.18b). The idea of using this gaming environment was to help children develop gross motor planning and coordination skills and learn these skills through entertainment.

In another study, researchers (Bhattacharya et al. 2015) designed Kinect-based activities in classroom settings for children with autism. The idea was to engage these children in movement-related activities and encourage peer interaction. Here, the researchers designed three motion-related activities, such as *game*, *free-form interaction*, and *interactive storytelling*. As regards the *game*, the task was to catch objects while scoring points. The user was free to choose his representation (live image or a skeleton image) on the screen in a way the user would like to see himself or herself on the screen. Additionally, the user could choose the background, such as jungle, space, etc. accompanied by individual soundtracks. Virtual objects appeared randomly on the screen. The task required the player to reach out to the object and touch it thereby scoring points. While one virtual object was touched, it was replaced by another object appearing randomly at another location.

For the *free-form interaction*, the screen display reflected the player's body and movements of the player. The player was free to choose representation of his or her choice along with background scenery. For representation, the available options were skeleton figure, iron man, princess, etc. For the background, the options were white screen, underwater scene, jungle scene, etc. This was designed as a single and multiplayer activity.

For the *interactive story*, still images of a story plot were projected on the screen. The task required the players to make gestures or movements so as to animate elements of the story as displayed on the screen. Additionally, soundtracks were added so as to make the task interesting. The story and the associated audio would stop for the player to make the necessary gesture. The Kinect sensor would wait to sense whether the necessary gesture was made by the player. Once the correct movement was done by the player, both the animation and the audio would resume again.

4.3.3.5.2   Wii-Assisted AR for Exergaming

Besides the Kinect-based exergaming platform, there is another exergaming platform. This is Wii Nintendo (Nintendo Inc., Kyoto, Japan) integrated with the virtual environment to offer AR-based gaming environment. However, the amount of energy expenditure during exergaming might be a toned down version of that with the Kinect-assisted exergaming solution since this uses upper body or limb movement ability as opposed to full body movement as in the case of Kinect-assisted exergaming (Smallwood et al. 2012). Still the Wii, Nintendo-based, cost-effective solution can be used to offer a three-dimensional spatial interaction for the purpose of gaming. Use of Wii Nintendo has been reported to cause more energy expenditure in a gaming scenario than that with sedentary games (Graves et al. 2008).

Nintendo Wii (from Nintendo of America, Inc., Redmond, WA) can offer an interactive gaming interface that focuses on fitness, motor skills, and eye–hand coordination (Getchell et al. 2012). Added to walking and running, the researchers included three Wii-based games, namely Wii Sport, Wii Fit, and Dance Dance Revolution (DDR). The Wii Sport was set to the beginner level. Here, the participants were asked to participate in various sports, such as tennis, bowling, boxing, baseball, etc. The Wii Fit was adjusted to the intermediate level. In this, the participants were asked to perform various fitness exercises, such as soccer heading, yoga move, torso twisting, etc. Based on how a participant performed in the Wii Sport and Wii Fit, the types of music and challenge level were chosen for the DDR. The video game-based DDR involved one to use rhythm and perform dance. In this, the participant was asked to stand on a platform and move his or her feet to touch various musical and visual cues, thereby generating music. Results indicated that the participants with autism spent maximum energy while walking, followed by running, followed by playing the DDR, followed by participating in Wii Fit that was in turn followed by Wii Sport.

4.3.4   Mixed Reality (MR) for Individuals with Autism

Mixed Reality comes at the intersection of human, computer, and environment. This can lead to a blending of the physical world with the digital world. The term, Mixed Reality was coined by Paul Milgram and Fumio Kishino (1994). At one extreme is Virtual Reality that occludes one's view by offering a digital experience. On the other extreme is the Augmented Reality that superimposes graphical representation on imagery of physical objects. Unlike Virtual Reality and Augmented Reality, the Mixed Reality preserves the experience of the physical world for the user while replacing the physical objects with digital representation. The Mixed Reality (MR) platform finds its place in applications relevant for children with autism and can play a key role in education, social behaviour training, etc. in the near future.

4.3.4.1   MR for Coaching Teachers Involved in Behavior-Related Training of Children with Autism

Children with autism are often characterized by social, communication, and behavioural problems. This in turn often makes teaching these children very complex (Ben Itzchak et al. 2008). Frequently, the behavioural problems, such as aggression, self-injurious behaviour, etc., can make it challenging for the teachers involved in special education schools to teach and manage them (Sullivan and Bradshaw 2012). Evidence-based intervention is powerful. But few teachers might have necessary training to use these techniques for addressing behaviour problems in the classroom (Shyman 2012). Additionally, given the unique demands of the children with autism and autism being a spectrum disorder, effective addressing of the behavioural deficits of multiple children at the same time at school might be challenging for the teachers. Thus, researchers (Pas et al. 2016) have proposed the use of Mixed Reality (MR) for training the teachers in addressing the behavioural deficits of the target group.

The researchers (Pas et al. 2016) have proposed the use of TeachLivE™ that is a Mixed Reality simulator to help teachers in learning new skills followed by immediate feedback, essential for effective teaching of skills (Dieker et al. 2008). Here, the teacher can interact with five simulated student avatars that can display animation and possess unique personalities. The behaviour of each virtual student could be modified based on the needs and each student could reciprocate to the teacher (having physical presence) in their individualized manner. Such training can help the teacher to get new insights and experience in classroom teaching.

4.3.4.2   MR-Based Games for Teaching Social Skills to Children with Autism

The literature review indicates that properly designed games can not only offer entertainment, but also show promise in skill learning that can be motivating (Gee 2007). It is well known that the children with autism have difficulties with verbal and non-verbal communication and interacting with their social partners (Gutstein et al. 2002). Additionally, these children prefer structured information and predictability that is referred to as 'static system' by researchers (Gutstein et al. 2002). In contrast, 'fluid system' is one that has a flow of novel information and is often referred to when we consider real-life interaction. Games can be a sort of a bridge in between the two systems since games can offer an avenue for goal-directed learning in which one can explore and experiment different options (Hoffmann 2009). This can be beneficial for students with autism.

Use of Situated Multimedia Arts Learning Lab (SMALLab) can offer such game-based learning scenarios enabled with Mixed Reality (Tolentino et al. 2009). One of the research studies (Tolentino et al. 2010) have used SMALLab to develop a collaborative learning environment in which children with autism can learn to interact by asking for help from a social partner. This game offered a physical environment in which students can move about and interact with digitized versions of robots accompanied with sound and images. This game featured images of discs lying on the floor. As the student moved, a robot followed the student and picked up the discs from the floor. The teacher had the freedom to sabotage the robot when the robot demonstrated peculiar actions, such as spinning around on its own, emitting sounds, etc. so as to give the impression that it has stopped working. To resume the task of collecting the discs, the student was expected to ask for help from the teacher. In turn, the teacher repaired the robot and the student again resumed taking the robot along with him or her for collecting the discs (projected as images). The game ended when all the discs were collected by the robot.

4.3.4.3   MR for Subject-Specific Training

Autism spectrum disorder is a neurodevelopmental disorder in which these children tend to become confused in real-life scenarios due to excessive noise, colours, and stimuli (Parés et al. 2005). Thus, exposing them to simulated scenarios where the level of information and variations can be controlled while maintaining attributes of the physical world can offer a good training platform. In such a case, Mixed Reality can be useful. For example, while teaching the concepts in a specific subject matter, MR can offer the learners with the feeling of embodiment while being immersed in the simulated world.

Researchers (Birchfield et al. 2008) have been exploring the use of MR in teaching concepts related to a particular subject matter, such as earth sciences to individuals. Here, the researchers have used *River City* (Ketelhut 2007) that is a multi-user simulated environment to teach children the concepts behind transmission of diseases. The *River City* comprised of a river that flowed through different terrains with water, air, and insects being responsible for the transmission of a disease. The students felt themselves to be embedded in the *River City* world in which they could interact with others, e.g. fellow avatars, avatars serving the role of facilitators, and experienced the auditory and visual stimuli associated with that world. The participants were free to take complex decisions, such as using virtual microscopes to study the water samples while discussing and sharing the possible solutions for addressing the issue of disease transmission.

4.4 Summary

In this chapter, I have introduced the readers to the various advantages offered by Virtual Reality (VR)-based applications to various stakeholders, such as the children with autism, the families of these children, the therapists, and last but not the least the designers. Subsequently, I have presented valuable information on the different types of VR-based platforms that can be used for intervention. Specifically, I have given detailed information on VR presented on a 2D screen of the computer monitor, immersive VR, Augmented (Virtual) Reality, and Mixed (Virtual) Reality. While describing each of these types of VR, I have informed the reader on the different applications that can be used for skill learning by individuals with autism. Thus, different examples focusing on learning of skills related to navigation, social communication, phobia, safety, pretend play, exergaming, shopping, daily living, self-awareness, imitation, etc. have been discussed while these have been applied by different investigators.

This chapter looks at the different aspects of the computer-based simulated worlds with a bird's-eye view mostly from the user's perspective. In the next chapter, I will present in-depth information on some of the design perspectives while considering interface design, adaptive switching of tasks of varying challenges, etc. with examples as far as social communication for these children is concerned.

References

Abbott BB, Badia P (1986) Predictable versus unpredictable shock conditions and physiological measures of stress: a reply to Arthur. Psychol Bull 100:384–387

Adjorlu A, Hoeg ER, Mangano L (2017) Daily living skills training in virtual reality to help children with autism spectrum disorder in a real shopping scenario. In: 2017 IEEE International Symposium on Mixed and Augmented Reality Adjunct Proceedings, pp 294–302

Ai-Lim Lee E, Wong KW, Fung CC (2010) How does desktop virtual reality enhance learning outcomes? A structural equation modeling approach. Comput Educ 55:1424–1442

Altanis G, Boloudakis M, Retalis S, Nikou N (2013) Children with motor impairments play a kinect learning game: first findings from a pilot case in an authentic classroom environment. Interact Des Arch 19:91–104

Bai Z, Blackwell A, Coulouris G (2015) Using augmented reality to elicit pretend play for children with autism. IEEE Trans Vis Comput Graph 21(5):598–610

Bandini LG, Gleason J, Curtin C, Lividini K, Anderson SE, Cermak SA, Maslin M, Must A (2012) Comparison of physical activity between children with autism spectrum disorders and typically developing children. Autism 17(1):44–54

Baron-Cohen S (1987) Autism and symbolic play. Br J Dev Psychol 5:139–148

Barsalou LW, Wiemer-Hastings K (2005) Situating abstract concepts. In: Pecher D, Zwaan RA (eds) Grounding cognition. Cambridge University Press, New York

Ben Itzchak E, Lahat E, Burgin R, Zachor AD (2008) Cognitive, behavior, and intervention outcome in young children with autism. Res Dev Disabil 29:447–458

Bergeron B (2006) Developing serious games (game development series)

Bernard-Opitz V, Sriram N, Nakhoda-Sapuan S (2001) Enhancing social problem solving in children with autism and normal children through computer-assisted instruction. J Autism Dev Disord 31(4):377–384

Bhattacharya A, Gelsomini M, Fuster PP, Abowd GD, Rozga A (2015) Designing motion-based activities to engage students with autism in classroom settings. In: IDC '15, 21–25 June 2015, Medford, MA

Birchfield D, Mechtley B, Hatton S, Thornburg H (2008) Mixed-reality learning in the art museum context. In: Proceedings of ACM SIG Multimedia, Vancouver, Canada, October–November 2008

Bozgeyikli E, Raij A, Katkoori S, Dubey R (2016) Locomotion in virtual reality for individuals with autism spectrum disorder. In: SUI'16, 15–16 October, Tokyo

Broun TL (2004) Teaching students with autistic spectrum disorder to read: a visual approach. Teach Except Child 36(4):36–40

Buckner RL, Carroll DC (2007) Self-projection and the brain. Trends Cogn Sci 1(2):49–57

Casas X, Herrera G, Coma I, Fernández M (2012) A Kinect based augmented reality system for individuals with autism spectrum disorders. In: Proc. GRAPP/IVAPP 2012, SciTePress, pp 240–246

Casasanto D (2009) Embodiment of abstract concepts: good and bad in right- and left-handers. J Exp Psychol Gen 138(3):351–367

Catherine T, Roy E (2003) Visual teaching strategies for children with autism. Early Child Dev Care 173(4):425–433

Chamberlain RS, Herman BH (1990) A novel biochemical model linking dysfunctions in brain melatonin, proopiomelanocortin peptides, and serotonin in autism. Biol Psychiatry 28 (9):773–793

Chen C-H, Lee I-J, Lin L-Y (2016) Augmented reality-based video-modeling storybook of non-verbal facial cues for children with autism spectrum disorder to improve their perceptions and judgments of facial expressions and emotions. Comput Hum Behav 55:477–485

Cihak DF, Moore EJ, Wright RE, McMahon DD, Gibbons MM, Smith C (2016) Evaluating augmented reality to complete a chain task for elementary students with autism. J Spec Educ Technol 31(2):99–108

Cohen S (1998) Targeting autism: what we know, don't know, and can do to help young children with autism. University of California Press, Berkley, CA

Colzato LS, van Leeuwen PJA, van den Wildenberg WPM, Hommel B (2010) DOOM'd to switch: superior cognitive flexibility in players of first person shooter games. Front Cogn 1:8

Corbett BA, Schupp CW, Levine S, Mendoza S (2009) Comparing cortisol, stress and sensory sensitivity in children with autism. Autism Res 2(1):39–49

Cromby JJ, Standen PJ, Brown DJ (1996) The potentials of virtual environments in the education and training of people with learning disabilities. J Intellect Disabil Res 40:489–501

Crozier S, Sileo N (2005) Encouraging positive behaviour with social stories. Teach Except Child 37(6):26–31

Dautenhahn K (1999) Robots as social actors: aurora and the case of autism. In: Proceedings Third Cognitive Technology Conference CT'99, August, San Francisco

Dettmer S, Simpson R, Myles B, Gantz J (2000) The use of visual supports to facilitate transition of students with autism. Focus Autism Other Dev Disabil 15(3):163–169

Dieker LA, Hynes MC, Hughes CE, Smith E (2008) Implications of mixed reality and simulation technologies on special education and teacher preparation. Focus Except Child 40(6):1–20

Dunn W, Brown C (1997) Factor analysis on the sensory profile from a national sample of children without disabilities. Am J Occup Ther 51(7):490–495

Eycke KDT, Müller U (2015) Brief report: new evidence for a social-specific imagination deficit in children with autism spectrum disorder. J Autism Dev Disord 45(1):213–220

Finkelstein SL, Nickel A, Barnes T, Suma EA (2010) Astrojumper: designing a virtual reality exergame to motivate children with autism to exercise. In: IEEE Virtual Reality, 20–24 March 2010, Waltham, MA, pp 267–268

Garner M, Mogg K, Bradley BP (2006) Orienting and maintenance of gaze to facial expressions in social anxiety. J Abnorm Psychol 115(4):760–770

Gee JP (2007) Good video games + good learning: collected essays on video games, learning, and literacy. P. Lang, New York

Getchell N, Miccinello D, Blom M, Morris L, Szaroleta M (2012) Comparing energy expenditure in adolescents with and without autism while playing Nintendo®Wii™ games. Games Health J 1 (1):58–61

Gjevik E, Eldevik S, Fjæran-Granum T, Sponheim E (2011) Kiddie-SADS reveals high rates of DSM-IV disorders in children and adolescents with autism spectrum disorders. J Autism Dev Disord 41:761–769

Graves L, Stratton G, Ridgers ND, Cable NT (2008) Energy expenditure in adolescents playing new generation computer games. Br J Sports Med 42(7):592–594

Gutstein S et al (2002) relationship development intervention with young children social and emotional development activities for Asperger syndrome, autism, PDD, and NDL. Jessica Kingsley Publishers, London

Halabi O, El-Seoud SA, Alja'am J, Alpona H, Al-Hemadi M, Al-Hassan D (2017) Design of immersive virtual reality system to improve communication skills in individuals with autism. IJET 12(05):50–64

Herrera G, Jordan R, Gimeno J (2006) Exploring the advantages of augmented reality for intervention in ASD. In: Proceedings of the World Autism Congress, South Africa

Herrera G, Alcantud F, Jordan R, Blanquer A, Labajo G, Pablo CD (2008) Development of symbolic play through the use of virtual reality tools in children with autistic spectrum disorders. Autism 12(2):143–157

Hillman CH, Belopolsky AV, Snook EM, Kramer AF, McAuley E (2004) Physical activity and executive control: implications for increased cognitive health during older adulthood. Res Q Exerc Sport 75(2):176–185

Hinkley T, Teychenne M, Downing KL, Ball K, Salmon J, Hesketh KD (2014) Early childhood physical activity, sedentary behaviors and psychosocial well-being: a systematic review. Prev Med 62:182–192

Hodgdon L (2000) Visual strategies for improving communication: practical supports for school and home. Quirk Roberts, Troy, MI

Hoffmann L (2009) Learning through games. Commun ACM 52(8):21–22

Inman DP, Loge K (1995) Demonstrating and evaluating a virtual reality training program for teaching mobility skills to orthopedically impaired children. In: Third Annual International Conference on Virtual Reality and Persons with Disabilities, San Francisco, August 1995

Iseminger SH (2009) Keys to success with autistic children: structure, predictability, and consistency are essential for students on the autism spectrum. Teach Music 16(6):28

Ivey JK (2004) What do parents expect?: a study of likelihood and importance issues for children with autism spectrum disorders. Focus Autism Other Dev Disabil 19(1):27–33

Jarrold C, Boucher J, Smith PK (1996) Generativity deficits in pretend play in autism. Br J Dev Psychol 14(3):275–300. https://doi.org/10.1111/j.2044-835X.1996.tb00706.x

Jones RA, Downing K, Rinehart NJ, Barnett LM, May T, McGillivray JA et al (2017) Physical activity, sedentary behavior and their correlates in children with autism spectrum disorder: a systematic review. PLoS One 12(2):e0172482. https://doi.org/10.1371/journal.pone.0172482

Joshi G, Petty C, Wozniak J, Henin A, Fried R et al (2010) The heavy burden of psychiatric comorbidity in youth with autism spectrum disorders: a large comparative study of a psychiatrically referred population. J Autism Dev Disord 40:1361–1370

Kavanaugh RD, Harris PL (1994) Imagining the outcome of pretend transformations: assessing the competence of normal and autistic children. Dev Psychol 30:847–854

Kenny MC, Bennett KD, Dougery J, Steele F (2013) Teaching general safety and body safety training skills to a Latino preschool male with autism. J Child Fam Stud 22(8):1092–1102

Ketelhut DJ (2007) The impact of student self-efficacy on scientific inquiry skills: an exploratory investigation in River City, a multi-user virtual environment. J Sci Educ Technol 16(1):99–111

Kreibig SD (2010) Autonomic nervous system activity in emotion: a review. Biol Psychol 84 (3):394–421

Kuriakose S, Lahiri U (2017) Design of a physiology-sensitive VR-based social communication platform for children with autism. IEEE Trans Neural Syst Rehabil Eng 25(8):1180–1191. https://doi.org/10.1109/TNSRE.2016.2613879

Kushki A, Drumm E, Mobarak MP, Tanel N, Dupuis A, Chau T, Anagnostou E (2013) Investigating the autonomic nervous system response to anxiety in children with autism spectrum disorders. PLoS One 8(4):e59730

Kushki A et al (2015) A Kalman filtering framework for physiological detection of anxiety-related arousal in children with autism spectrum disorder. IEEE Trans Biomed Eng 62(3):990–1000

Laky V, Lanyi CS (2003) To develop virtual reality worlds for treating agoraphobia and acrophobia. In: Proc. VRIC Virtual Reality International Conference, Laval, 2003, pp 127–133

Lang R, Koegel L, Ashbaugh K, Regester A, Ence W, Smith W (2010) Physical exercise and individuals with autism spectrum disorders: a systematic review. Res Autism Spectr Disord 4 (4):565–576

LaViola JJ (2000) A discussion of cybersickness in virtual environments. ACM SIGCHI Bull 32 (1):47–56

Leslie AM (1987) Pretence and representation: the origins of "theory of mind". Psychol Rev 94:412–426

Leyfer OT, Folstein SE, Bacalman S, Davis NO, Dinh E et al (2006) Comorbid psychiatric disorders in children with autism: interview development and rates of disorders. J Autism Dev Disord 36:849–861

Lind SE, Williams DM (2012) The association between past and future oriented thinking: evidence from autism spectrum disorder. Learn Motiv 43:231–240

Lind SE, Williams DM, Raber J, Peel A, Bowler DM (2013) Spatial navigation impairments among intellectually high-functioning adults with autism spectrum disorder: exploring relations with theory of mind, episodic memory, and episodic future thinking. J Abnorm Psychol 122 (4):1189–1199

Lord C, Rutter M, DiLavore P, Risi S (2001) Autism diagnostic observation schedule-WPS edition. Western Psychological Services, Los Angeles, CA

Maskey M, Lowry J, Rodgers J, McConachie H, Parr JR (2014) Reducing specific phobia/fear in young people with autism spectrum disorders (ASDs) through a virtual reality environment intervention. PLoS One 9:e100374. https://doi.org/10.1371/journal.pone.0100374

Matsentidou S, Poullis C (2014) Immersive visualizations in a VR Cave environment for the training and enhancement of social skills for children with autism. In: 2014 International Conference on Computer Vision Theory and Applications (VISAPP), Lisbon, 2014, pp 230–236

Mattila M-L, Hurtig T, Haapsamo H, Jussila K, Kuusikko-Gauffin S et al (2010) Comorbid psychiatric disorders associated with Asperger syndrome/high-functioning autism: a community- and clinic-based study. J Autism Dev Disord 40:1080–1093

Mayes SD, Calhoun SL, Aggarwal R, Baker C, Mathapati S et al (2013) Unusual fears in children with autism. Res Autism Spectr Disord 7:151–158

Mazzone L, Postorino V, De Peppo L, Fatta L, Lucarelli V, Reale L, Giovagnoli G, Vicari S (2013) Mood symptoms in children and adolescents with. Autism Spectr Disord Res Dev Disabil 34 (11):3699–3708

McComas J, Mackay M, Pivik J (2002) Effectiveness of virtual reality for teaching pedestrian safety. Cyberpsychol Behav 5(3):185–190

Milgram P, Kishino F (1994) A taxonomy of mixed reality visual displays. In: IEICE Transactions on Information Systems, Vol E77-D, No. 12, December 1994

Must A, Phillips SM, Curtin C, Anderson SE, Maslin M, Lividini K, Bandini LG (2013) Comparison of sedentary behaviors between children with autism spectrum disorders and typically developing children. Autism 18(4):376–384

Nally B, Houlton B, Ralph S, Mudford O (2000) Researches in brief: the management of television and video by parents of children with autism. Autism 4(3):331–338

Norbury CF, Brock J, Cragg L, Einav S, Griffiths H, Nation K (2009) Eye movement patterns are associated with communicative competence in autistic spectrum disorders. J Child Psychol Psychiatry 50(7):834–842

Orth T (2003) Diet & nutrition: teaching anyone to cook for themselves. Except Parent 33(2):30–34

Pan CY (2008) Objectively measured physical activity between children with autism spectrum disorders and children without disabilities during inclusive recess settings in Taiwan. J Autism Dev Disord 38(7):1292–1301

Parés N, Masri P, van Wolferen G, Creed C (2005) Achieving dialogue with children with severe autism in an adaptive multisensory interaction: the "MEDIATE" project. IEEE Trans Vis Comput Graph 11(6):734–742

Park D, Youderian P (1974) Light and number: ordering principles in the world of an autistic child. J Autism Child Schizophr 4:313–323

Parsons S, Mitchell P (2002) The potential of virtual reality in social skills training for people with autistic spectrum disorders. J Intellect Disabil Res 46:430–443

Parsons TD, Rizzo AA (2008) Affective outcomes of virtual reality exposure therapy for anxiety and specific phobias: a meta-analysis. J Behav Ther Exp Psychiatry 39:250–261

Parsons S, Mitchell P, Leonard A (2004) The use and understanding of virtual environments by adolescents with autistic spectrum disorders. J Autism Dev Disord 34(4):449–466

Parsons S, Mitchell P, Leonard A (2005) Do adolescents with autistic spectrum disorders adhere to social conventions in virtual environments? Autism 9:95–117

Pas ET, Johnson SR, Larson KE, Brandenburg L, Church R, Bradshaw CP (2016) Reducing behavior problems among students with autism spectrum disorder: coaching teachers in a mixed-reality setting. J Autism Dev Disord 46(12):3640–3652

Paynter J, Peterson CC (2013) Further evidence of benefits of thought-bubble training for theory of mind development in children with autism spectrum disorders. Res Autism Spectr Disord 7 (2):344–348

Peeters T (1997) Autism: from theoretical understanding to educational intervention. Singular Publishing Group, San Diego, CA

Perner J, Frith U, Leslie AM, Leekam SR (1989) Exploration of the autistic child's theory of mind: knowledge, belief and communication. Child Dev 60:689–700

Piaget J (1952) The origins of intelligence in children. Norton, New York

Pirker J, Gütl C, Belcher JW, Bailey PH (2013) Design and evaluation of a learner-centric immersive virtual learning environment for physics education. In: SouthCHI 2013, LNCS 7946, pp 551–561

Pot-Kolder R, Veling W, Counotte J, van der Gaag M (2018) Anxiety partially mediates cybersickness symptoms in immersive virtual reality environments. Cyberpsychol Behav Soc Netw 21(3):187–193

Prior M, Hoffman W (1990) Neuropsychological testing of autistic children through an exploration with frontal lobe tests. J Autism Dev Disord 20:581–590. https://doi.org/10.1007/BF02216063

Raj P, Oza P, Lahiri U (2017) Gaze-sensitive virtual reality based social communication platform for individuals with autism. IEEE Trans Affect Comput 9(4):450–462. https://doi.org/10.1109/TAFFC.2016.2641422

Rebenitsch L, Owen C (2016) Review on cybersickness in applications and visual displays. Virtual Reality 20(2):101–125

Ricciardi JN, Luiselli JK, Camare M (2006) Shaping approach responses as intervention for specific phobia in a child with autism. J Appl Behav Anal 39(4):445–448

Rizzo A, Difede J, Rothbaum BO, Daughtry JM, Reger G (2013) Virtual reality as a tool for delivering PTSD exposure therapy. In: Post-traumatic stress disorder: future directions in prevention, diagnosis, and treatment. Springer, New York, NY

Rose D, Foreman N (1999) Virtual reality. Psychologist 12(11):550–554

Rusch FR, Cimera RE, Millar DS et al (2002) Crossing streets: a K–12 virtual reality application for understanding knowledge acquisition. [On-line]. http://archive.ncsa.uiuc.edu/Edu/RSE/VR/trivr.html

Rutherford MD, Rogers SJ (2003) Cognitive underpinnings of pretend play in autism. J Autism Dev Disord 33(3):289–302

Rutter M, Le Couteur A, Lord C (2003) Autism diagnostic interview-revised. Western Psychological Services, Los Angeles, CA

Saiano M, Pellegrino L, Casadio M, Summa S, Garbarino E, Rossi V, Agata DD, Sanguineti V (2015) Natural interfaces and virtual environments for the acquisition of street crossing and path following skills in adults with autism Spectrum disorders: a feasibility study. J Neuroeng Rehabil 12:17

Salvatore S (1974) The ability of elementary and secondary school children to sense oncoming car velocity. J Saf Res 6:118–125

Sandles S (1975) Children in traffic. Elek, London

Sandlund M, Hoshi K, Waterworth EL, Hager-Ross C (2009) A conceptual framework for design of interactive computer play in rehabilitation of children with sensorimotor disorders. Phys Ther Rev 14(5):348–354

Schreibman L, Koegel RL (2005) Training for parents of children with autism: pivotal responses, generalization, and individualization of interventions. In: Hibbs ED, Jensen PS (eds) Psychosocial treatments for child and adolescent disorders: empirically based strategies for clinical practice. American Psychological Association, Washington, DC, pp 605–631

Self T, Scudder RR, Weheba G, Crumrine D (2007) A virtual approach to teaching safety skills to children with autism spectrum disorder. Top Lang Disord 27(3):242–253

Sherman WR, Craig AB (2003) Understanding virtual reality: interface, application, and design. Morgan Kaufmann Publishers, Boston

Shyman E (2012) Teacher education in autism spectrum disorders: a potential blueprint. Edu Train Autism Dev Disabil 47:187–197

Silver M, Oakes P (2001) Evaluation of a new computer intervention to teach people with autism or Asperger syndrome to recognize and predict emotions in others. Autism 5(3):299–316

Sinha P, Kjelgaard MM, Gandhi TK, Tsourides K, Cardinaux AL, Pantazis D, Diamond SP, Held RM (2014) Autism as a disorder of prediction. Proc Natl Acad Sci USA 111(42):15220–15225

Smallwood SR, Morris MM, Fallows SJ, Buckley JP (2012) Physiologic responses and energy expenditure of Kinect active video game play in schoolchildren. Arch Pediatr Adolesc Med 166 (11):1005–1009

Smith IM, Bryson SE (1994) Imitation and action in autism: a critical review. Psychol Bull 116 (2):259–273

Stahmer AC, Collings NM, Palinkas LA (2005) Early intervention practices for children with autism: descriptions from community providers. Focus Autism Other Dev Disabil 20:66–79

Stahmer AC, Schreibman L, Cunningham AB (2011) Toward a technology of treatment individualization for young children with autism spectrum disorders. Brain Res 1380:229–239

Standen PJ, Brown DJ (2005) Virtual reality in the rehabilitation of people with intellectual disabilities: review. Cyberpsychol Behav 8(3):272–282; discussion 283–288

Steinhauer GD (1984) Preference for predictable small rewards over unpredictable larger rewards. Psychol Rep 54:467–471

Strickland D (1997) Virtual reality for the treatment of autism. In: Riva G (ed) Virtual reality in neuropsycho-physiology. IOS Press, Amsterdam, pp 81–86

Strickland D, Mesibov GB, Hogan K (1996) Two case studies using virtual reality as a learning tool for autistic children. J Autism Dev Disord 26:651–659

Strickland DC, McAllister D, Coles CD, Osborne S (2007) An evolution of virtual reality training designs for children with autism and fetal alcohol spectrum disorders. Top Lang Disord 27 (3):222–237

Sullivan T, Bradshaw CP (2012) Introduction to the special issue of behavioral disorders: serving the needs of youth with disabilities through school-based violence prevention efforts. Behav Disord 37(3):129–132

Summers J, Tarbox J, Findel-Pyles RS, Wilke AE, Bergstrom R, Williams WL (2011) Teaching two household safety skills to children with autism. Res Autism Spectr Disord 5:629–632

Swettenham J (1996) Can children with autism be taught to understand false belief using computers? J Child Psychol Psychiatry 37(2):157–165

Tartaro A, Cassell J (2007) Using virtual peer technology as an intervention for children with autism. In: Lazar J (ed) Towards universal usability: designing computer interfaces for diverse user populations. Wiley, Chichester

Taylor M (2013) Transcending time, place, and/or circumstance: an introduction. In: Taylor M (ed) The Oxford handbook of the development of imagination. Oxford University Press, New York, NY, pp 3–10

Tentori M, Escobedo L, Balderas G (2015) A smart environment for children with autism. IEEE Pervasive Comput 14:42–50

Thomdyke PW, Hayes-Roth B (1982) Differences in spatial knowledge acquired from maps and navigation. Cogn Psychol 14:560–589

Tiator M, Kose O, Wiche R, Geiger C, Dorn F (2018) Trampoline jumping with a head-mounted display in virtual reality entertainment. In: Intelligent Technologies for Interactive Entertainment, pp 105–119

Tolentino L et al (2009) Teaching and learning in the mixed reality science classroom. J Sci Educ Technol 18:6

Tolentino L, Savvides P, Birchfield D (2010) Applying game design principles to social skills learning for students in special education. In: FDG 2010, 19–21 June, Monterey, CA

Tolman EC (1948) Cognitive maps in rats and men. Psychol Rev 55:189–208

Trepagnier CY, Sebrechts MM, Finkelmeyer A, Stewart W, Woodford J, Coleman M (2006) Simulating social interaction to address deficits of autistic spectrum disorder in children. Cyberpsych Behav 9(2):213–217

Tsai YF, Viirre E, Strychacz C, Chase B, Jung TP (2007) Task performance and eye activity: predicting behavior relating to cognitive workload. Aviat Space Environ Med 78(Suppl 1): B176–B185

Vafadar M (2013) VR: opportunities and challenges. History of VR and its use in medicine

Volkmar FR, Wiesner LA (2009) A practical guide to autism: what every parent, family member and teacher needs to know, 1st edn. John Wiley and Sons, Inc., Hoboken, NJ, 610 pp. ISBN 978-0-470-39473-1

Wellman HM, Baron-Cohen S, Caswell R, Gomez JC, Swettenham J, Toye E, Lagattuta K (2002) Thought-bubbles help children with autism acquire an alternative to a theory of mind. Autism 6 (4):343–363

Williams DM (2010) Theory of own mind in autism: evidence of a specific deficit in self-awareness? Autism 14(5):474–494. ISSN 1461-7005

Witwer AN, Lecavalier L (2010) Validity of comorbid psychiatric disorders in youngsters with autism spectrum disorders. J Dev Phys Disabil 22:367–380

Chapter 5
Design of Virtual Reality-Based Applications in Autism Intervention

5.1 Introduction

In the previous chapter, I have presented different types of computer-based applications, particularly considering the umbrella term Virtual Reality (VR) ranging from 2D VR presented on a 2D computer monitor, Augmented (Virtual) Reality, Immersive (Virtual) Reality, and Mixed (Virtual) Reality. Also, by now, you know the use of the VR-based solutions in addressing skill deficits of children with autism. Additionally, you are aware of the numerous advantages of using VR particularly for individuals with autism. The VR can serve as an excellent tool in the hands of the interventionists for offering different training scenarios to the users, controllable levels of challenge based on an individual's specific abilities, adaptive skill learning environment, etc. Researchers around the globe have been using VR for individuals with autism while offering them tasks that can contribute to improvement in social communication, emotion recognition, joint attention, etc. Offering skill training in at least some of these core deficit areas is important since the children with autism are often characterized by deficit in making socially appropriate reciprocation while carrying out back-and-forth communication with social partners, understanding facial emotional expressions, following the gaze of a social partner to triangulate to an object of interest through shared attention, etc. In this chapter, I will present detailed information on the building of the various components, such as Graphical User Interface, virtual characters, individualized and adaptive feedback of 2D VR-based applications.

In fact, nowadays, investigators have extensively explored the applicability of VR in the areas of entertainment, skill learning, intervention, etc. while using different types of VR-enabled platforms. Among the different types, I choose the VR-based applications that can be presented on 2D computer screen since this can offer a cost-effective platform and can be deployed even in homes without extensive costs of setting it up. Specifically, it does not need extensive hardware such as dedicated external peripheral devices as needed in the case of Augmented Reality, Immersive

© Springer Nature Switzerland AG 2020   131
U. Lahiri, *A Computational View of Autism*,
https://doi.org/10.1007/978-3-030-40237-2_5

Reality, etc. With computers (desktop and laptop) being available at various homes and special needs schools, even in countries with developing economy, using computers to present 2D VR-based training scenarios for the children can be a feasible solution. Thus, in this chapter, I will present detailed information on the building of the various components of such 2D VR-based applications (termed as VR *henceforth*).

Specifically, I am going to focus on the various design considerations of VR such as design of graphical user interface (GUI) of the stimulus, the adaptive nature of the VR-based application, and the design of the avatars that serve as virtual characters. While describing these aspects, I will consider specific application areas as examples.

5.2   Design Considerations in Using Virtual Reality (VR) to Address Deficits in Social Interaction Skills

Children with autism are often characterized by deficits in social interaction and communication that can be attributed to their restricted patterns of interest and behaviour (APA 2000) and difficulties in carrying out complex fluid reciprocal social interactions (Carpenter et al. 2002) along with infrequent engagement in social interactions (APA 1994). Again, autism being a spectrum disorder, success of an intervention depends on the individualization of services to a great extent. Thus, the use of appropriately individualized, intensive behavioural and educational intervention is on the rise with the intervention being tuned to address specific deficits, such as social communication deficit of individuals with autism (NRC 2001) in an individualized manner. In spite of the benefits of availing appropriately designed intervention services, there are barriers with regard to accessibility of such specialized services for the stakeholders. For example, the first limitation is restricted availability of trained interventionists that is particularly true in developing countries like India. The second limitation is the modality used for delivery of intervention services. Specifically, such specialized intervention requires long hours of one-on-one sitting of the interventionist with the child that can be challenging, given the limited trained resources. Often, the one-on-one intervention sessions are very expensive (Ganz 2007; Goodwin 2008) that in turn restricts its accessibility to the common man. The exorbitant cost can be both direct and indirect in nature. Specifically, the direct cost can be the charges needed to avail the specialized services from the interventionist. On the other hand, the indirect cost can be in terms of the caregiver not being able to earn his or her own living since he or she has to invest his or her time in taking care of the child, accompanying the child to the clinic, etc. Given these barriers, investigators are exploring the potential of technology to offer services that can increase the accessibility coupled with intensive and individualized intervention (Goodwin 2008). Amidst the different types of technology-assisted systems, here, I present the role of VR that can offer a skill learning environment for a child in an individualized manner.

With desktop VR, one can easily design communication scenarios set in social contexts. With computing power becoming cheaper, use of desktop VR can ensure the ease of accessibility and affordability (Cobb et al. 1999) to the user. Also, researchers have shown that desktop VR can be effectively experienced by a user (Parsons and Mitchell 2002). Again, instead of games that are only entertaining, one can design serious games while using VR-based softbots, e.g. avatars acting as facilitators. Using VR, the avatars can be made to blink, speak in a lip-synched manner, perform gestures, move dynamically in the VR-based environment, etc. that can appear realistic to the user. Exposure to such a training environment can promote communication-related skill learning in the individual with autism. The communication-related skill can have various aspects such as initiating a conversation, ability to reciprocate in a bidirectional conversation, etc. While an individual is exposed to such a VR-based training environment, the VR-based system can provide valuable information on specific aspects of the deficit of an individual (such as those related to social communication) to the caregivers and clinicians. This information, in turn, can help them to modify the intervention paradigm. Also, such a system can keep a record of the improvement in performance of the learner (say a child with autism), thereby helping the caregivers and clinicians to monitor the progress (in skill learning) of the learner.

Here, I present details on one of the research studies with a focus on the design of a VR-based social communication task platform that exposed a child to bidirectional social communication with an avatar (that is a virtual peer) embedded in different social contexts (Lahiri et al. 2013). The social communication task platform comprised of various components such as

1. User Interface for task presentation
2. Bidirectional conversation
3. Task performance evaluator
4. Logic for going to the next task

5.2.1 User Interface for Task Presentation

A python-based Vizard software from WorldViz LLc. was used to design the user interface. This software comes with a limited number of VR-based characters (i.e. the avatars) and a limited repository of social scenes. Thus, researchers have designed their own avatars and incorporated social scenes in the training platform based on the requirement.

As far as the design of avatars (3D humanoid characters projected on a 2D computer monitor) was concerned, 2D photographs with front and side views of human faces along with necessary textures (to cause variations in the VR-based characters) were used. These photographs were mounted on the head skeleton of avatars available with the Vizard software. The avatar heads were then associated with the torso of the 3D characters. Subsequently, the animations were programmed in the Vizard environment. The avatars were capable of blinking, speaking in a lip-synched manner, and demonstrating gestures, such as raising arms for pointing towards an object of interest and moving dynamically within the VR environment.

The avatars were programmed to narrate their personal experience to the user while being embedded in relevant social contexts. For narration, a database of stories was created. As far as the social contexts were concerned, a repository of contexts depicting scenes relevant to the experience was created that was narrated by the avatar in the form of a story. While presenting these contexts, the VR environment was modulated to depict scenes that were relevant to the narration by the avatar. The avatar's narration was based on a variety of relevant topics, e.g. a sport of choice, events related to a special day in the life, trip in the countryside with friends, etc. For each social context, the avatar was programmed to make a one-on-one interaction with the user (i.e. a child with autism).

As an example, let us consider an avatar narrating his experience of travel to a beach in which he introduced the viewer (i.e. a participant with autism) to the sea beach, glimpses of situations on the sea beach, etc. As can be seen from Fig. 5.1a, an avatar shared his experience of visiting a sea beach and describing the beautiful terrain comprising of the rocks swept by sea water at regular intervals while standing in such a context as projected by the VR-based environment. During the narration, the avatar shared his experience of the various events that he witnessed on the sea beach. For example, the avatar described the chairs that were laid down on the beach (Fig. 5.1b) for the tourists to enjoy the sunbath. During this time, the VR environment portrayed such a situation to the user. Again, while the avatar walked along the sea beach, he shared his experience of witnessing the sunset (Fig. 5.1c) towards the end of his tour with the VR scene depicting such a situation to the user. While the avatar (embedded in the VR environment) described his personal experience related to a social context to the users, the users could view the avatar from the first-person perspective that is in line with research on social anxiety and social conventions (Pereira et al. 2009).

5.2.2   Bidirectional Conversation

An important component of social communication is the ability to interact with and reciprocate to a social partner. Thus, after the avatar finished presenting the task, the user was exposed to a bidirectional communication interface. This interface was designed to be menu driven. The bidirectional communication interface appeared with menu choices for a user to choose his or her question meant to be asked to the avatar. The menu choices were offered so as to serve as an (1) easy reference to the individual with autism for communication and (2) give a structure to the two-way communication. Thus, to every piece of information that the participant was expected to extract from the avatar, the participant could refer back to the possible options presented on the communication interface.

The task required the participant to extract a piece of information from the avatar. The piece of information was categorized as (1) 'Benign', (2) 'Projected Contingent'

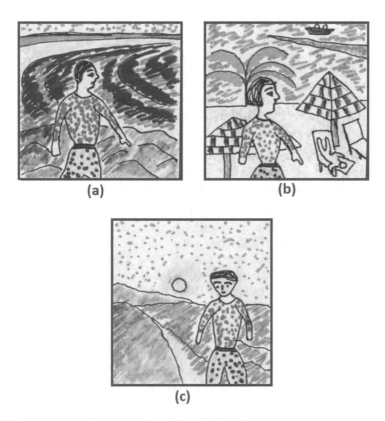

Fig. 5.1 An avatar narrating his tour experience during his visit to a sea beach while describing the (**a**) rocky beach, (**b**) chairs meant for sunbath, and (**c**) view of the sunset

(targeting information beyond what was described by the avatar during the task presentation), and (3) 'Sensitive' (one related to the personal feeling). Additionally, based on the category of the information to be extracted by the participant from the avatar, the tasks were designed to belong to three interaction challenge levels (i.e. difficulty levels of interaction) such as 'Easy', 'Medium', and 'High'. Again, extraction of information belonging to the three categories (as mentioned above) needed the participant to go through different lengths of conversation threads. By conversation thread, I mean, two-way reciprocation during avatar–participant communication. Added to narrating his experience, the avatar also served as a facilitator giving necessary hints to the participant in case of discrepancy in the use of the conversation threads. Here, I discuss the three challenge levels of interaction.

5.2.2.1   'Easy' Level of Interaction

For an 'Easy' interaction, a user was expected to retrieve a 'Benign' piece of information from the avatar. Specifically, this information was meant to be context-relevant and based on the content of the narration by the avatar. The number of conversation threads was limited to asking a few, such as three questions to the avatar. Also, the order of asking such questions was important. The idea was that the user should learn to carry on such a conversation with a social partner while using

1. Introduction (with the social communicator), followed by
2. Asking about the topic of the conversation, and finally by
3. Asking about the avatar's overall feeling related to the situation

Children with autism face milestones in initiating any conversation. One of the best ways to initiate a social communication is to introduce oneself while displaying proper gestures. The avatar started by nodding his head or by waving his hand and telling his name as an introductory gesture. Thus, while using the bidirectional communication interface, the participant was also expected to start with a brief introduction about himself or herself. This was followed by his or her comments and questions posed to the avatar with an intention to extract a piece of information from the avatar.

For example, once an avatar finished describing his experience of a rugby game during the task presentation, the user was asked to extract a 'Benign' piece of information, e.g. the avatar's experience regarding his first rugby match (Fig. 5.2). As can be seen from Fig. 5.2, the bidirectional response interface had three options addressing aspects of introduction, topic of the context being narrated by the avatar, and that related to the avatar's feeling (presented in randomized order), respectively. In this example, the third option was related to the introduction, the first option was on the topic of the conversation, and the second option was related to the avatar's personal feeling related to playing rugby.

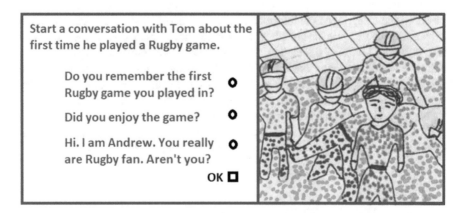

Fig. 5.2 An example of 'Easy' level of interaction with bidirectional response interface

The avatar was programmed to enact the roles of a social partner and also as a facilitator. For example, if a user chose the third option at first, then the avatar enacted the role of a social partner by reciprocating back accordingly, such as the avatar said that

Yes, you are correct. I like Rugby and I am a big fan of Rugby.

In contrast, if the user chose any other option before choosing the third option, then the avatar played the role of a facilitator by offering hints to the user regarding the fact that one needs to finish the introduction first before going ahead with the social conversation. In such a case, the avatar told

It looks like we do not know each other. May be we should introduce ourselves first.

Subsequently, if the participant chose the first option, then the avatar reciprocated by saying

Yes, I do. The first Rugby match that I played was on the day I finished the final exam of my 6th standard class.

In case, the participant chose the second option before the first option, the avatar, serving as a facilitator said

Are you referring to any particular match that I played?

Finally, when the participant chose the second option, the avatar said

Yes, I enjoyed the first Rugby match. After that I decided not to miss any Rugby game.

5.2.2.2 'Medium' Level of Interaction

For Medium difficulty, a user was expected to retrieve a 'Projected Contingent' piece of information from the avatar. Specifically, this information was meant to be context-relevant. Additionally, this was intended to get additional information that may be superficially connected with the contents of narration by the avatar. In other words, it needed one to extend the thought while knitting some facts before asking a question. The conversation threads featured five questions that were needed to be asked by the user. Also, the order of asking such questions was important.

1. First an introductory question was to be asked. This was to be followed by
2. Asking about the topic of the conversation, given that the information to be extracted was projected contingent.
3. Then one can probe more on the topic of the discussion. Based on the communicator's response regarding the topic of the conversation, one
4. Could continue with asking about the particulars within that topic, followed by some description of that topic. Finally, one could
5. Conclude by asking about the overall impression of the topic of the conversation.

Let us consider an example as shown in Fig. 5.3 in which an avatar narrated her experience of a busy day spent on the weekend with her friends while she went to a

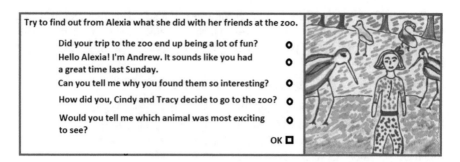

Fig. 5.3 An example of 'Medium' level of interaction with bidirectional response interface

movie theatre, shopping mall, followed by a tour of a zoo. The user was asked to find out some more information regarding how the avatar spent her time at the zoo that was not touched upon by the avatar during the task presentation (that is the narration). As can be seen from Fig. 5.3, the bidirectional response interface had five options presented in a randomized order. In this case, the second option was meant for an introduction. If a participant chose the second option first, then the avatar said

Yes, Andrew. Last Sunday, I had a great time with my friends.

In case a participant did not choose the second option at first, then the avatar reciprocated while offering hints to the participant that they need to introduce themselves first. Since the topic of the information needed to be retrieved was related to the zoo, one could be expected to choose the fourth option. Thus, if the participant chose the fourth option, the avatar responded by saying

Well, all of us really like animals, particularly seeing them in their own habitats. Plus, this zoo is the only place in America where people can see animals from China.

In case, instead of choosing the fourth option, the participant chose any other option, then the avatar said

I visited movie theatre, shopping mall and the zoo with my friends. It seems that you are interested to hear more about the zoo. Is it?

In turn, the user was expected to choose the fifth option while focusing on the particulars of the topic as mentioned by the avatar. Thus, the avatar responded by saying

I found the blue Pandas very interesting. I could see a mother and her child Panda.

In case, the participant missed choosing the fifth option, the avatar was programmed to say

It seemed to me that you were interested in hearing about animals that I found interesting during my trip to the zoo.

After the avatar narrated briefly on the particulars, the participant was expected to probe a bit deeper to know some more details on the topic by choosing the third option. In such a case, the avatar responded by saying

Surely. The blue Pandas are dangerous animals, but they do not look like harmful.

However, in case the third option was not chosen by a participant, then the avatar said

Since I was sharing with you my experience of seeing the blue Pandas, I thought that you would like to hear more about them. Isn't it?

Finally, the conversation ended with the participant asking the avatar regarding her overall experience of the trip to the zoo by choosing the first option. In response, the avatar said

Yes, it was real fun visiting the zoo. It seems like I cannot wait to visit the zoo again.

Thus, the avatar enacted the roles of a peer responding to the questions asked by a participant and also like a facilitator while giving necessary hints to the participant so as to foster a free flow of thoughts during the conversation.

5.2.2.3   'High' Level of Interaction

For the High level of interaction, a user was expected to retrieve a 'Sensitive' piece of information from the avatar. By sensitive topic, I mean any topic that relates to some unpleasant feeling or experience of the social peer that one would not generally like to share during a social conversation. Each conversation thread had seven questions (presented in a randomized order) that were meant to be asked by a participant. Also, the order of asking these questions was important. In this,

1. The conversation began with a basic introduction by the social communicator, similar to that in the Easy and Medium levels of difficulty.
2. Since the topic of discussion was a sensitive one, it expected one to ask permission from the social communicator before going ahead with the topic as a good social gesture.
3. Based on the communicator's response regarding his or her willingness to share his or her thoughts on a sensitive topic, one could start with mentioning a brief on the topic followed by asking a broad question related to the sensitive topic.
4. Upon getting a positive response from the communicator, one could probe a bit more to get some details on the topic.
5. If the communicator responded properly, then one might proceed to get information (on a broader level) on any memory or event related to the sensitive topic. Then one
6. Could delve a bit deeper to get finer aspects of the memory or event associated with the topic.
7. Finally, the conversation ended with the communicator's views or thoughts regarding the sensitive topic.

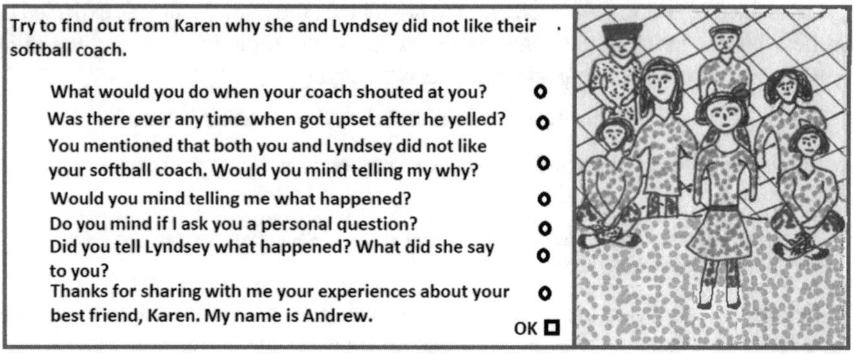

> **Try to find out from Karen why she and Lyndsey did not like their** ·
> **softball coach.**
>
>   What would you do when your coach shouted at you?   O
>   Was there ever any time when got upset after he yelled?   O
>   You mentioned that both you and Lyndsey did not like
>   your softball coach. Would you mind telling my why?   O
>   Would you mind telling me what happened?   O
>   Do you mind if I ask you a personal question?   O
>   Did you tell Lyndsey what happened? What did she say   O
>   to you?
>   Thanks for sharing with me your experiences about your   O
>   best friend, Karen. My name is Andrew.   OK ☐

Fig. 5.4 An example of 'High' level of interaction with bidirectional response interface

For example, let us consider a scenario in which an avatar is narrating an experience of playing softball with her friend and mentions having an unpleasant experience while interacting with the coach. The system prompted the participant to get information on a sensitive topic such as the relation of the avatar with the softball coach. The participant was expected to start the conversation with the introductory session by choosing the seventh option (Fig. 5.4). In response, the avatar reciprocated by saying

Hello Andrew. Hope you liked to hear that.

In case the participant chose any other option at first, the avatar said

It looks like we do not know each other. May be we should introduce ourselves first.

Since, the topic of the conversation has been a sensitive one, the participant was expected to first ask permission while following social etiquettes by choosing the fifth option. To this the avatar said

No, I would not mind. Please go ahead.

If instead of choosing the fifth option, a participant chose any other option, then the avatar said

It seemed that you were interested to hear about some of my experiences related to the playing of softball that I was mentioning during my narration. Isn't it?

After hearing that the social communicator found it okay to discuss on the sensitive topic, the participant was expected to choose the third option. Specifically, the participant described the context briefings followed by asking about the sensitive topic.

Yes. I did not like the softball coach since he had a bad habit of shouting at the players.

In case the participant chose any other option instead of the third option, then the avatar said

Is it regarding the softball coach that you wanted to hear?

Once the avatar responded while mentioning the reason such as the coach having a bad habit of shouting at the players, the participant was expected to choose the first option. The idea was to get specific details on the topic. To this, the avatar said

I used to feel very nervous and kept quiet. Then, I used to try not to make any mistake again.

In case the first option was not chosen and instead any other option was chosen by the participant, then the avatar said

Was it about my feeling in general, when the coach used to shout?

Having heard that the avatar used to feel nervous about hearing the coach shout, the participant was expected to probe deeper by asking about any specific event or incident by choosing the second option. To this, the avatar would say

Yes. I remember that. That was the day before the semi-final match in March 2010, when he shouted at me.

In case the participant missed the second option, then the avatar said

Were you interested to hear about any incident related to the coach shouting at me?

Once the avatar responded stating the unpleasant event that she experienced, the participant was expected to probe a bit deeper into the specific event by choosing the fourth option. To this, the avatar would say

No. I would not mind. I was trying to pitch the ball, but I'm not the best pitcher. The coach shouted at me with a red face, saying, Hey, don't you know how to throw?

If the participant missed choosing the fourth option, the avatar said

Were you interested to hear about the details of the specific incident in which the coach shouted at me?

Finally, the participant was expected to conclude the conversation by choosing the sixth option. To this, the avatar responded by saying that

Yes. I shared this with my friend. My friend made me feel better, because she agreed that he had been mean. Then, she helped me practice pitching and the next day I was a lot better. Our coach didn't shout at me then!

Thus, similar to the roles enacted by the avatars during the 'Easy' and 'Medium' levels of interaction, in the case of 'High' level of interaction, the avatar was capable of playing both the roles of a facilitator and a social partner involved in a back-and-forth communication with the participant. Whenever the participant missed adhering to the correct order in which the questions were needed to be asked, the avatar provided the participant necessary hints to facilitate the conversation.

5.2.3 Task Performance Evaluator

The maximum scores that could be achieved while using the bidirectional social conversation module were 30, 50, and 70 for Easy, Medium, and High levels of interaction difficulty, respectively. Additionally, the system allotted a penalty factor for an irrelevant choice made by a participant while interacting with the avatar (an irrelevant choice referred to one not maintaining the expected order of asking the questions to the avatar). Also, the performance score was labelled as *Adequate* (in case the total score was $\geq 70\%$) or *Inadequate* (otherwise).

5.2.3.1 Task Performance Evaluation for the Easy Level of Interaction

Let us consider a task in the Easy level of interaction as shown in Fig. 5.2. In this case, three choices were presented to the participant. The maximum achievable score was 30 points with 10 points being allotted to each of the three relevant choices being made.

While considering Fig. 5.2, the third option, related to the introduction phase, was expected to be the first to be chosen by a participant while interacting with the avatar. This was to be followed by the second option in which the participant was expected to ask about the topic of the conversation that was on the playing of rugby. Finally, the participant was expected to choose the first option in which the participant wanted to know the overall feeling that the avatar had about the specific topic, i.e. his experience of his first rugby match that he had played. Thus, while conversing with the avatar, if the participant chose the third option the first in the first attempt, then the participant scored 10 points. However, if the participant chose the first or the second option the first time, followed by choosing the third option the second time, the system allotted 6 points to the participant. Else, if the participant chose the third option the third time (i.e. on the third attempt), then the system allotted 2 points to the participant. The system was programmed to permit a participant to make 2 irrelevant choices for the Easy level of interaction.

Again, an option that had been chosen by a participant could not be chosen again. In other words, no backtracking was allowed. Again, if the participant chose the third option the first, followed by choosing the first option that in turn was followed by choosing the second option (Fig. 5.2), then the participant scored 30 points (out of the maximum score of 30 points). In other words, the performance score was 100 (or 100%) that was considered as *Adequate*.

However, let us consider a case in which if the participant chose the correct option (third option here) in the second attempt, followed by choosing the first option that in turn was followed by choosing the second option, then the participant scored 22 points (out of a maximum possible score of 30 points). Thus, the performance score was approximately 73 (or, 73%) that was also considered as *Adequate*.

Again, let us consider the worst case in which if a participant started the interaction by choosing the first option followed by choosing the second option that in turn was followed by choosing the third option (the relevant choice in this case), the system allotted 2 points to the participant. Subsequently, if the participant chose the second option followed by choosing the first option, then the participant could score 6 points with the cumulative score being 2 points + 6 points = 8 points. Finally, while finishing the interaction, if the participant chose the second option, the system allotted the participant 10 points with the total cumulative score being 2 points + 6 points + 10 points = 18 points (out of a maximum score of 30 points). In other words, the participant's performance score was 60% that was considered as *Inadequate*.

5.2.3.2   Task Performance Evaluation for the Medium Level of Interaction

Now let us consider a task in the Medium level of interaction (Fig. 5.3). In this case, the maximum score that could be achieved was 50 points with 10 points being allotted to each relevant choice.

While considering Fig. 5.3, a participant was expected to choose the second option (related to the introduction) at first, followed by choosing the fourth option (related to the topic of the conversation), followed by choosing the fifth option (related to the particulars of the topic of conversation), followed by choosing the third option (related to the specifics of the topic of conversation), and finally followed by choosing the first option (related to the overall reactions on the topic of the conversation). Thus, if a participant made relevant choices for each option, then the participant scored 50 points (out of the maximum possible score of 50 points, i.e. 100%). This was considered as the *Adequate* performance.

Again, let us consider a case in which if a participant started the conversation by choosing the second option in the third attempt, then the system allotted a score of 2 points. If this was followed by the participant choosing the fourth option in the second attempt, then the system allotted the participant 6 points, with the cumulative score being 2 points + 6 points = 8 points. Then, if this was followed by the participant choosing the fifth option in the first attempt, then the allotted score was 10 points with the cumulative score being 8 points + 10 points = 18 points. Again, if this was followed by the third option being chosen in the first attempt, the system allotted 10 points and the cumulative score was 18 points + 10 points = 28 points. Finally, if the participant chose the first option in the first attempt, the system allotted 10 points to the participant with the cumulative score being 28 points + 10 points = 38 points. Thus, the participant could score 38 points (out of a maximum of 50 points) that amounted to 76% and that was considered as *Adequate* performance.

Again, let us consider a scenario in which a participant chose the second option in the third attempt, thereby scoring 2 points. Then, if the participant chose the fourth option in the third attempt, then the system allotted 2 points with the cumulative score being 2 points + 2 points = 4 points. Again, if the participant chose the fifth option in the third attempt while scoring 2 points for this option with the cumulative score being 4 points + 2 points = 6 points. Then, if the participant chose the third option in the second attempt, the system awarded the participant with 6 points with the cumulative score being 6 points + 6 points = 12 points. Finally, if the participant chose the first option, the system allotted 10 points for this option choice with the cumulative score being 12 points + 10 points = 22 points out of a maximum of 50 points (i.e. 44%) that was labelled as *Inadequate* performance.

5.2.3.3   Evaluation of Task Performance for High Level of Interaction

Let us consider a task in the High level of interaction difficulty (Fig. 5.4). In this case, the maximum score that could be achieved was 70 points with 10 points being allotted to each relevant choice.

While considering Fig. 5.4, a participant was expected to choose the seventh option (related to the introduction) at first, followed by choosing the fifth option (related to asking permission to discuss a personal issue that was a sensitive topic of discussion), followed by the third option (related to approaching the sensitive topic in a broader sense), followed by the first option (related to the specific details on the sensitive topic), followed by the second option (related to a memorable event or incident connected with the sensitive topic), followed by choosing the fourth option (related to the details on the memorable event or incident connected with the sensitive topic), and finally followed by choosing the sixth option (related to the effects of the event on someone). Thus, if the participant chose all the relevant options in the first attempt, then the total performance score of the participant was 70 (that is 100%). This was considered to be *Adequate* performance.

Let us consider an example in which a participant missed choosing the relevant options in the first attempt for the first few questions being asked to the avatar. For example, say a participant was able to choose the seventh option in the third attempt. Here, the allotted performance score was 2 points. Again, this were followed by the participant choosing the fifth option in the third attempt, thereby scoring 2 points. Thus, the cumulative performance score was 2 points + 2 points = 4 points. If this was followed by the participant choosing the third option in the second attempt, then the system gave 6 points and the cumulative performance score was 4 points + 6 points = 10 points. In turn, if this was followed by choosing the first option by the participant in the first attempt, then the participant was awarded 10 points, with the cumulative performance score being 10 points + 10 points = 20 points. Again, if this was followed by choosing the second option in the first attempt, then the awarded score was 10 points with the cumulative performance score being 20 points + 10 points = 30 points. After this, if the participant chose the fourth option in the first attempt, then the performance score was added by 10 points with the cumulative performance score being 30 points + 10 points = 40 points. Lastly, if the participant was left with the sixth option that the participant chose in the first attempt, then 10 points were awarded on this response. Thus, the cumulative performance score was 40 points + 10 points = 50 points (out of a maximum of 70 points). Thus, the percentage performance score was approximately 71% that was labelled as *Adequate* performance.

Again, let us consider a scenario in which a participant chose the seventh option in the third attempt causing him to score 2 points. Following this, if the participant chose the fifth option in the third attempt, then this resulted in 2 points to be allotted.

This caused the cumulative task performance score to be 2 points + 2 points = 4 points. If this was followed by a participant choosing the third option in the third attempt, then 2 points were awarded for this. The cumulative score was 4 points + 2 points = 6 points. Then, if the participant chose the first option in the third attempt, the cumulative score was 6 points + 2 points = 8 points. After this, if the participant chose the second option in the third attempt, then the cumulative score was 8 points + 2 points = 10 points. Again, if this was followed by the participant choosing the fourth option in the second attempt thereby scoring 6 points on this response, the cumulative score was 10 points + 6 points = 16 points. Finally, being left with the sixth option, if the participant chose the sixth option in the first attempt, then the cumulative score was 16 points + 10 points = 26 points (out of a maximum of 70 points) for this task. Thus, the percentage performance score was approximately 37% that was considered as *Inadequate* performance.

Based on whether the task performance score was *Adequate* or *Inadequate*, the system decided to switch the tasks that were presented to the participants.

5.2.4   Logic for Task Switching (for Presenting the Next Task)

Based on how a participant performed a task, his task performance score was labelled either as *Adequate* or *Inadequate*. After this, the system switched to a new task being presented by using a State Machine representation. The State Machine (Booth 1967) can be used to represent a behaviour model that consists of a finite number of states, transition between the states, and the corresponding actions when certain conditions are met. In the present case, the number of states was three with the first one representing the Easy, the second indicating the Medium, and the last one representing the High level of interaction difficulty (as mentioned above). The transition was in terms of switching to a next task based on the conditions such as the performance score being *Adequate* or *Inadequate*.

For example, based on a participant's performance while choosing the questions of the conversation thread (as mentioned above), the participant's performance score was evaluated and labelled as being *Adequate* (performance score being ≥70%) or *Inadequate* (otherwise). Thus, there were two task switching conditions, namely

1. Condition1 (i.e. COND1) for *Adequate* performance
2. Condition2 (i.e. COND2) for *Inadequate* performance

Based on the participant's performance, the tasks were offered by the system using a state machine based task switching rationale (Fig. 5.5). If COND1 was satisfied, the system offered tasks of increased challenge. Vice versa was the case if COND2 was satisfied.

Let us consider an example in which a participant was interacting with a VR-based task belonging to the Easy level of interaction. If the participant's performance score was *Adequate* (i.e. COND1), then the system presented the participant with a task belonging to higher challenge, i.e. one belonging to Medium

Fig. 5.5 State Machine representation for offering tasks of varying difficulty (Easy, Medium, and High interaction level). Note: COND1 and COND2 indicate Condition1 and Condition2, respectively

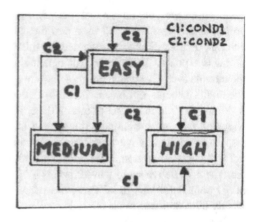

level of interaction. However, if the participant achieved an *Inadequate* score (i.e. causing COND2 to be satisfied), then the Easy level of interaction being a task belonging to the lowest challenge level, the system will present a task belonging to the same difficulty level (i.e. Easy level of interaction) with the hope that the participant could perform better next time. Again, if the participant was executing a task belonging to the Medium level of interaction, then for *Adequate* performance (COND1), the system presented a task of High level of interaction. Else, if the performance was *Inadequate* (COND2), then the system presented a task of reduced challenge that is one belonging to the Easy level of interaction. Finally, if the participant was interacting with a task belonging to the High level of interaction, then for *Adequate* performance (i.e. COND1), the system presented a task belonging to the same difficulty level, i.e. a task belonging to the High level of interaction difficulty. This was because the High level of interaction difficulty was the highest challenge level in the present example. However, if the performance score was *Inadequate* (i.e. COND2), then considering that the task belonging to the High level of interaction was difficult for the participant, the system presented a task of lower challenge, i.e. one belonging to the Medium level of interaction difficulty.

To summarize, the VR-based system was sensitive to the participant's task performance score, thereby challenging the user with tasks of higher difficulty in case of *Adequate* performance.

5.2.5   An Experimental Investigation

Using the above-mentioned system, an experimental study was designed for individuals with autism.

5.2.5.1   Participants

High-functioning teenaged individuals (ASD1–ASD8) with autism (Mean (SD) = 15.76 (1.89) years) were recruited to participate in this study. The participants were tested using Peabody Picture Vocabulary Test (PPVT) (Dunn and Dunn 1997) test scores, Social Responsiveness Scale (SRS) (Constantino 2002), Social Communication Questionnaire (SCQ) (Rutter et al. 2003a), Autism Diagnostic Observation Scale-Generic (ADOS-G) (Lord et al. 2000), and the Autism Diagnostic Interview-Revised (ADI-R) (Rutter et al. 2003b). On an average, the scores were Mean (SD) = 112 (20.51) for PPVT score, 77.25 (13.28) for SRS score, 17.5 (5.57) for SCQ score, 9 (2) for ADOS-G, and 43.33 (16.26) for ADI-R score.

The PPVT score can be considered as a proxy for IQ testing because of the high correlation of PPVT with standard IQ testing scales such as the Wechsler Intelligence Scale for Children (Bee and Boyd 2004). From the PPVT scores, we can say that on an average, the participants with autism were non-retarded. As far as the SRS scores were concerned, three participants with ASD were in the Mild to Moderate range and the rest was in the Severe range. Again, considering the SCQ scores, the participants met the autism cut-offs. Also, the ADOS-G and ADI-R scores indicated that the participants had autism.

5.2.5.2   Procedure

Each volunteer was expected to participate for 1.5 h in this study. The participant was introduced to the system followed by an initial adaptation phase. Then the signature of consent or assent forms was administered. This was in turn followed by the Virtual Reality-based task lasting for approximately 30 min. In the introductory phase, the experimenter introduced herself and described the experimental set-up to the participant, followed by using a visual schedule to narrate what the participant was expected to do. In the adaptation phase, the participant was asked to interact with demo sessions comprising of computer-based tasks. During the administration of the signing of consent/assent forms, the participants or their caregivers gave consent to take part in the study. Also, the participants were told that they were free to leave the study in case they felt uncomfortable while interacting with the computer-based tasks.

The experimental set-up comprised of a task computer that was operated in the master mode and a secondary monitor operated in the slave mode. The task computer was used to present the VR-based tasks to the participants. The signals from the task computer were routed to a second monitor for the experimenter, a therapist, and the participant's caregiver to observe how the task progressed. Finally, once the participants expressed their willingness to start interacting with the VR-based tasks, the experimenter started the computer-based tasks.

The task began with an initial instruction screen that showed the participant the steps required to carry out the task. This was followed by an avatar narrating his or her experience to the participant while moving dynamically inside the VR scene depicting context-relevant situation. After this, the participant was asked to find out a piece of information from the avatar. Subsequently, a menu-driven bidirectional communication interface was presented to the participant. The participants could select one option choice at a time with the help of the computer mouse. To every question or comment from the participant, the avatar responded back. After a few back-and-forth interactions between the participant and the avatar, the task ended.

As mentioned before, the system offered tasks belonging to three difficulty levels, namely Easy, Medium, and High. Also, within the task execution, there was a baseline stage followed by the main task execution stage. During the baseline stage, a participant was exposed to one task from each challenge level. During the baseline stage, the avatar did not enact the role of a facilitator, thereby not giving hints on the correct option choice that the participant was expected to make. Subsequently, the challenge level in which the participant scored the highest was chosen for the main task execution stage. This was done to find out the challenge level that best suited the participant so that the main task execution stage can start with that challenge level in an individualized manner. Thus, for example, if a participant scored 100% in Easy, 60% in Medium, and 40% in High challenge level, then the system offered tasks belonging to the Easy difficulty level to start with during the main task execution stage. However, if the participant scored 100% in Easy, 100% in Medium, and 60% in High difficulty level, then a task belonging to the Medium difficulty level was chosen to start with during the main task execution stage. During the main task execution stage, the avatar enacted the role of a facilitator so as to facilitate the participant to walk through the conversation threads in case the participant made irrelevant choices (while responding to the participant's question or comment using the bidirectional conversation interface).

5.2.6   Results

The acceptability of the system by the target population was first studied. This was followed by the analysis of the participants' task performance score.

5.2.6.1   Acceptability of the System

None of the participants left the tasks in the midway in spite of given an option to discontinue from the tasks in case one felt uncomfortable at any point during the task execution. An exit survey carried out at the end of the study revealed that all of them liked interacting with the VR-based social communication platform, particularly while using the bidirectional conversation interface. Also, they did not report any problem in understanding the stories narrated by the avatars during the task execution. When asked if they had any take-home lessons that they have learnt while interacting with the virtual classmates, all of them expressed that they learned that they should introduce themselves first while speaking with a peer the first time. Also, they inquired regarding future possibilities of exposure to the system. Thus, from this one can infer that such a system has potential to be accepted by the target population.

5.2.6.2   Task Performance

As far as the task performance was concerned, different participants interacted with the system in their own way. Figure 5.6 shows the performance of each participant.

It can be seen from Fig. 5.6 that ASD1, ASD5, and ASD6 interacted with tasks belonging to all the three difficulty levels during the main task execution stage. In contrast, ASD2, ASD7, and ASD8 started with a task belonging to the Medium interaction level during the main task execution stage. However, ASD3 and ASD4 started with a task in the High interaction level while executing the main task. Overall, the average minimum percentage performance score was 80%.

5.3   Feasibility of Virtual Reality to Address Deficit in Emotion Recognition Capability

It is well known that one's ability to extract socially relevant information from the communicator's face is one of the fundamental skills crucial to facilitate successful reciprocity during social communication (Trepagnier et al. 2002). An early deficit in such a skill may adversely affect one's development, and it is often a milestone faced by children with autism (Dawson 2008). This can be partially attributed to the children with autism exhibiting an atypical looking pattern with greater fixation towards non-social objects than the social stimuli, such as the faces of partners during social communication. Such a deficit can have a cascading effect that is manifested in terms of difficulty in interpreting a communicator's

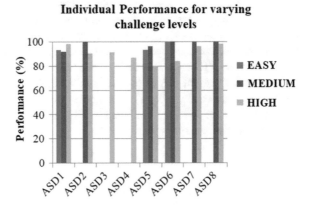

Fig. 5.6 An analysis of task performance of participants with autism

emotional expressions. The emotional expression can be manifested either verbally or non-verbally (such as through facial expression). The children with autism have a deficit in picking up non-verbal cues, such as emotional expression on the face of a social communicator. These children exhibit a tendency to particularly avoid the eye region of a social communicator, thereby failing to pick up some of the complex emotions of the partner during communication. Looking towards the eye region of a social communicator might be important for proper recognition of emotional expressions demonstrated by a social partner. Researchers have reported the dominance of gaze fixation towards different regions of one's face, such as eyes, mouth, etc. based on the facial emotional expression. For example, researchers such as Eisenbarth and Alpers (2011) have shown that typically developing individuals demonstrate the varying dominance of fixation on the eye and mouth regions, while scanning the face of a social communicator exhibiting different facial emotional expressions, such as afraid, angry, happy, neutral, and sad. Again, when one observes a communicator's face showing specific emotional expression, the phenomenon of imitation termed as mimicry (Canon et al. 2009) sets in as a result of emotional contagion (Moody et al. 2007). However, a quick and automatic imitation of emotional expression is seldom observed among children with autism (McIntosh et al. 2006) that in turn adversely affects their social communication.

Researchers have been examining the mechanism by which children with autism process social cues, particularly by reading the communicators' faces (Rutherford and Towns 2008; Jones et al. 2008). Such a deficit often leads to the children with autism displaying difficulties in social judgement that hampers lucidity in their reciprocation to carry out a social conversation along with context-irrelevant behaviour and lack of emotional reciprocity (Baron-Cohen et al. 1999; Carpenter et al. 2002). Additionally, these children exhibit increased engagement in non-social tasks (McGee et al. 1997; Sigman and Ruskin 1999) that often steals away their ability to pick up emotional cues from a social partner. Given these deficits, researchers have been focusing on ways to design affect-sensitive interactive skill training platforms with an aim to train the individuals with autism so that they can appropriately reciprocate after deciphering the emotional content.

Given the deficits of children with ASD related to an understanding of the facial emotional expressions of a social partner, researchers have been investigating the use of technology to develop skill training applications for these children. In fact, VR has been used by researchers to project social contexts along with virtual characters who can demonstrate context-specific emotional expressions. The flexibility in programming offered by VR can enable designers to offer such scenarios to the children with autism. Here, I present one of the research studies (Lahiri et al. 2011) that offered VR-based scenarios in which (1) virtual peers were programmed to display different facial emotional expressions followed by (2) participants being asked to recognize the facial emotional expressions.

5.3.1 VR-Based Tasks with Avatars Displaying Emotional Expressions

Both the presentation and understanding of context-relevant emotional expressions are important for having a lucid social communication. Using VR-based platform, it is easy to project 3D virtual humanoid characters (avatars *henceforth*) that can be capable of presenting context-relevant emotional expressions. Thus, avatars (male and female) were programmed in VR to display different facial emotional expressions, such as happy, angry, and neutral (as shown in Fig. 5.7, speaking in a lip-synched manner and blinking. The avatars' heads were created from 2D photographs of real individuals mounted on the head skeletons using 3DMeNow software. The different facial emotional expressions were programmatically created by using PeopleMaker software in which the morphs can be used in a calculated manner so as to control the intensity of the emotional expression. The avatar's eyes were programmed with a blink morph in which the avatar's eyes were alternately opened and closed so as to simulate random blinking every 1 and 2 s that is in line with the reports by Itti et al. (2003). As far as speaking was concerned, the avatars were programmed to speak in a lip-synchronized manner with pre-recorded audio files created with the help of typically developing individuals who were age-matched with the participant pool comprising of individuals with autism.

Additionally, the avatar was made to appear in a VR-based room environment, having photo frames displaying images of social contexts being narrated by the avatar. The avatar's narration comprised of different sections, namely introduction, contexts, and a conclusion. In the introduction section, the avatar mentioned his or her name along with a brief description on the contexts that he or she would like to narrate. For example, the avatar would say

Hi, I am Tom. I love watching sports and mostly these are outdoor sports.

Then, the avatar described his or her experience on three contexts, such as cricket, football, and hockey. The photo frame inside the VR-based room displayed a collage

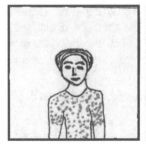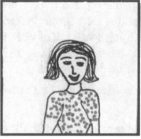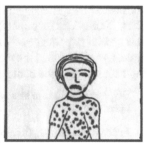

Fig. 5.7. Example of avatars displaying neutral (left), happy (middle), and angry (right) facial expression

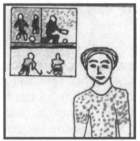 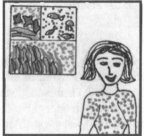 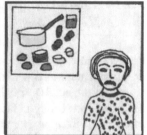

Fig. 5.8 Avatars with the photo frames depicting outdoor sports (left), sea world (middle), and food items (right)

of the snapshots of the narrated contexts (here the outdoor sports (Fig. 5.8)). Additionally, the avatar demonstrated context-relevant emotional expressions.

Each story narration (by the avatar) was approximately 3 min long. In each story, the avatar exhibited a specific emotional expression to capture the mood inherent in the content of the story. Again, care was taken that the avatar displayed one emotional expression throughout the narration. For example, if the avatar shared his experience of watching the cricket, football, and hockey, the narration was framed in a way that the avatar had similar experience, say, neutral experience for all the three outdoor sports. Thus, the avatar displayed neutral facial expression while narrating his experience to the participant. Again, let us consider a case in which the avatar expressed her interest in learning about sea creatures. However, her experience while visiting a water park (having various sea creatures) had been pleasant, then the avatar displayed happy emotional expression while narrating her experience to the participant. At the end of each story narrated by the avatar, the participant was asked to respond to questions based on the story content (context-relevant) and on the emotion (Emotion-Identification question) displayed by the avatar.

As far as the story content was concerned, care was taken that the topic of the question was mentioned at least five times in the narration by the avatar that is considered as sufficient for the information to be conveyed by the avatar (Jonides et al. 2008). The incorrect options were never spoken. For example, if the avatar narrated his experience of watching sports out of which he liked the cricket the most and thus he described the reasons behind his liking (in his narration) while mentioning about it, then the content-related question was

> I hope that you liked to hear my experience in watching outdoor sports. What is the sport that I like the most?

Each question had three options. For example, the option choices in the case of the narration on outdoor sports, e.g. cricket, football, and hockey, were

(a) *Cricket*
(b) *Snow scooting*
(c) *Badminton*

Each of the Emotion-Identification questions comprised of three options. Also, care was taken that the tone of the voice of the avatar was kept as neutral as possible so that the participants had to look at the faces of the avatars in order to correctly identify the emotions as exhibited by the avatars during the narration. An example of the Emotion-Identification question asked was

How did I feel while narrating my experience on the outdoor sports?

The response options were

(a) *Happy*
(b) *Angry*
(c) *Not Sure*

For each question, the participant was free to choose one of the three options. At the end of the study, the participants were asked about their impression on their interaction with the avatar (humanoid character, i.e. virtual peer). All the participants expressed that they liked interacting with the avatar. Also, they expressed that they did not face any difficulty in understanding the stories narrated by their virtual peers, or while responding to the questions asked by the avatar.

5.3.2 Methodology of the Experimental Investigation

This study had five VR-based social communication scenarios in which the virtual peers (i.e. the avatars) narrated their experience on different topics such as outdoor sports, travel, food, etc.

5.3.2.1 Experimental Set-Up

The experimental set-up comprised of a task computer and a second monitor. The task computer was a desktop computer, and it was placed on a table with a chair (meant for the participant) kept facing the table. The second monitor was kept away from the participant's view. This monitor was connected to the task computer. This monitor was used for the therapist and the caregiver to observe how the task progressed along with the responses of the participant to the questions asked by the avatar at the end of the narration. The experimental room was adequately lit. The study had ethical clearance.

5.3.2.2 Participant Characteristics

Six adolescents with autism (Mean (Standard Deviation) = 15.60 (1.27) years of age) volunteered for the study. All the participants had scored ≥80 on the Peabody Picture Vocabulary Test 3rd Edition (PPVT-III). The participants were tested for their autism-related measures. For this, their parent report was obtained on the Social Responsiveness Scale (SRS) and the Social Communication Questionnaire (SCQ). The SRS and SCQ scores of all the participants were found to be above the clinical thresholds.

5.3.2.3 Procedure

The study required a commitment of about 30 min from each participant. When the participant walked into the study room, the participant was asked to sit on a chair and the experimenter described the experimental set-up. Also, the participant was told that he or she was free to leave from the study at any time if he or she felt uncomfortable in interacting with the system. Further, each participant was told that he or she will meet virtual characters. The participants were asked to think of these virtual characters as their peers. They were told that the virtual peers will narrate their experience on topics of interest followed by asking questions to the participants. Also, they were told that the avatars would ask them questions that were relevant to the contexts being narrated by the avatars along with questions on how the avatars were feeling while narrating their experience.

5.3.3   Experimental Findings

5.3.3.1 Acceptability

In spite of being given the option of quitting from the study at any time if one felt uncomfortable, all the participants with autism completed the study. An exit survey was conducted after the experiment was over. It was found that all the participants liked interacting with the VR-based scenarios and did not face any problem in understanding the narrations of the virtual characters or in responding to the questions asked by their virtual peers. Also, most of them asked about future possibilities of interacting with the VR-based task environment. Thus, such a platform can have potential to be accepted by the target population.

5.3.3.2 Observations

All the participants were able to score almost 100% in the context-relevant questions indicating that they were paying attention while listening to the stories narrated by the avatars. As far as the Emotion-Identification questions were concerned, most of the participants were able to offer a correct response indicating that they were able to identify the expressions, except a few, who were confused in distinguishing the angry and happy expressions from neutral expression.

5.4   Role of Virtual Reality to Address Deficits in Joint Attention

In order to nurture a lucid social communication, it is essential for the communicators to have intact joint attention (JA *henceforth*) skill. The JA can be broadly categorized as initiating joint attention (IJA) and response to joint attention (RJA) (Mundy et al. 2009). The IJA refers to the process of initiating a cue intentionally so as to get the attention of a social partner to an object of interest. The RJA refers to the process of reciprocation to a cue being delivered by a social partner followed by attending to the cued object of interest. In other words, the RJA refers to the ability of an individual to pick up a cue prompted by a social partner and in turn follow the cue to attend to the prompted target of interest. If a social partner has cued by shifting gaze to prompt towards a target of interest, then the RJA can be considered as 'Looking where someone else is looking' (Sigman and Kasari 1995). For effective social communication, both the IJA and RJA are critical.

The administration of JA skill requires the use of both verbal and non-verbal cues prompting towards an object of interest while sharing attention with a social partner (Paparella et al. 2011). The verbal cue can be delivered using audio instructions. Again, the non-verbal modalities of offering JA cues can be eye gaze-based pointing, finger pointing gestures, etc. (Ferraioli and Harris 2011). In the eye gaze-based pointing, one changes the gaze orientation to point towards the target of interest. As far as the pointing gesture is concerned, one can use a raised arm with a pointed finger to direct towards the target of interest. One can also hold a pointer in the hand, such as a stick to point towards the object of interest. For example, a mother is trying to initiate a JA task by prompting her child to get a toy kept on a table. For this, the mother can use gaze-based cuing prompts by pointing her gaze towards the toy. In turn, she would expect that her child will respond to the JA task by following her gaze and look towards the toy (that is the object of interest) prompted by her. In case the mother finds that the child has failed to pick up her gaze cue, the mother might use other cues (that might be more informative for the child) such as finger-pointing gesture coupled with gaze cue and audio instruction to prompt the child to attend to the toy.

Generally, one's JA skill gets established during the early stages of development (Taylor and Hoch 2008). However, the evidence from the literature shows that children with autism are often characterized by limitations in JA skill (Sigman and Kasari 1995). In other words, these children often fail to exhibit IJA and RJA. Such deficits can have cascading effects, often manifested as a delay in language acquisition and social communication skills (Bono et al. 2004). Thus, it is crucial to address the JA skill deficit right from the early stages of development.

Some of the widely accepted conventional approaches are Pivotal Response Training (PRT), Physical Prompting, Fading Procedures, Parent tutoring, etc. (Bruinsma et al. 2004). Though these are promising (Meindl and Cannella-Malone 2011; Whalen and Schreibman 2003), yet the administration of these techniques is often costly and unaffordable for the masses since these need long hours of one-on-

one intervention (Chasson et al. 2007) and time from the therapist. Researchers have proposed VR-assisted platforms (Little et al. 2016; Caruana et al. 2017, 2018) for imparting JA skill training to individuals with autism.

5.4.1 VR-Based JA Task with Head Turn Being Used for Prompting

Let us consider a study by Little et al. (2016). This presents the design of a VR-based JA task environment in which an avatar had been used to administer JA task by using head turn-based cuing. The avatar cued towards any one of the two targets displayed on either side of the VR scene. The targets could be social, such as faces of individuals or non-social, such as images of buildings. Figure 5.9 shows a thematic representation. It can be seen from Fig. 5.9 that the avatar prompted a participant towards a target of interest by turning its head to point towards the target of interest. In this case, the avatar has turned its head with eyes oriented towards the left to point towards one of the faces or one of the houses ('target object'). The other image of the face or the house that the avatar had not prompted was considered as the 'non-target object'.

In this, both the participants with autism and typically developing (TD) children took part. Results indicate that the children with autism looked lesser towards the 'target object' as compared to that of their TD counterparts indicating that children with autism have a JA skill deficit. Such an observation might be attributed to the fact that the head of the avatar (used to prompt a target object) being a social stimulus might have posed difficulty for the child to follow the prompt delivered by the avatar. In contrast, the children with autism looked more often towards the 'non-target object' stimuli unlike the TD children. This might be because the non-target object did not have any social stimuli (such as the head of the avatar prompting towards the object) associated with it.

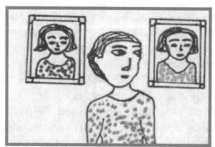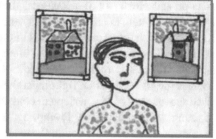

Fig. 5.9 Thematic representation of VR-based avatar-mediated JA task in which avatar has exhibited head turn

5.4.2   VR-Based JA Task with Gaze Cue Being Used for Prompting

Apart from the head turn, a prompting cue can be delivered with the help of gaze-based cuing. Again, in a particular task, it is important to understand the distinction between the intentional gaze cuing and unintentional eye movement of a social partner, such as in a search process. For establishing a JA bid successfully, one needs to understand the intention behind the gaze cue as issued by the social partner. This intention can be in the form of asking one to attend to a particular object in the visual scene.

The researchers such as Caruana et al. (2017) have studied this aspect of a JA task. In this, the researchers presented a VR-based JA task in which TD participants took part. An eye tracker (camera-based device) was used to pick up the participant's eye movement. In this study, the head of a person (an avatar) was used and the avatar's eye gaze could be oriented in different directions as needed. The avatar's head was positioned centrally between two rows of three houses each, one row above and the other below the avatar. Figure 5.10 shows a thematic representation. One row of houses had blue-coloured doors and the other row of houses had red doors. The task was to find a burglar who was hiding in one of the six houses. Here the avatar used gaze cue to administer the JA task. The tasks were designed as Search Tasks and NoSearch Tasks. In the Search Tasks, the participants were asked to search for the burglar by looking towards one row of houses while the avatar was responsible to search for the burglar by looking towards the other row of houses.

Fig. 5.10 Thematic representation of an avatar demonstrating gaze cue in a VR-based JA task

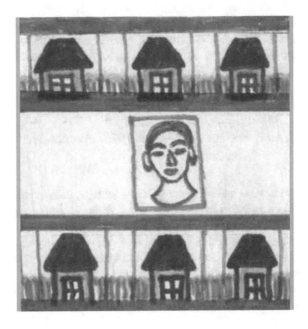

Also, both the participant and the avatar could see the interior of the houses upon fixating gaze on the doors of the houses only for the houses in the row that were allotted to them. While looking towards the houses allotted to him or her, the participant could not find the burglar in any of the houses, thereby giving the impression that the burglar was hiding in one of the houses in the row allotted for the avatar. Thus, the participant was asked to fixate on the face of the avatar. This was followed by the avatar displaying non-communicative eye moves while performing the search. Subsequently, the avatar displayed an intentional gaze-based cue towards a particular house. If the participant was able to understand the intention and moved his or her gaze to fixate on the house as cued by the avatar, then the burglar was captured. Again, in the NoSearch Task (similar to the Search Task), there was no search phase while responding to the joint attention (RJA). In other words, the component involving the monitoring of intention of a social partner was not there in this task. This study showed the efficacy of VR-based JA task platform to have a measurable influence on the one's JA behaviour.

Another study by Caruana et al. (2018) showed positive contributions of VR-based JA skill training of adults with autism. The same study, as mentioned above, was extended to incorporate both individuals with autism and the typically developing (TD) individuals. Results indicated that during the initial exposure, the participants with autism were able to interact with fewer trials as compared to their age-matched TD counterparts. This might infer that their speed of establishing a JA bid was much less as compared with that of their TD counterparts. However, on extended exposure to the VR-based JA skill training scenarios, the participants with autism performed better with the speed of response being nearly indistinguishable from that of the TD group. This shows that the VR-based JA task platform can be effectively used for offering JA skill training to the individuals with autism. Another important finding from this study was that the individuals with autism face difficulties in inferring the intention behind the gaze-based cue. This in turn can be attributed to their difficulty in establishing eye contact with a social partner that can be helpful in interpreting or understanding the action or intention of the partner.

5.4.3 VR-Based JA Task with Avatar-Mediated Hierarchical Prompting

In conventional observation-based settings, the therapist often changes the information content in the cuing message while administering the JA task. For example, while exposing a child to a JA task, the therapist might first use gaze-based prompting in which the therapist looks towards an object of interest and expect the child to follow her gaze and attend to the cued object. In case, the therapist finds that the child is unable to establish the JA bid, then the therapist might increase the prompting information by adding more information to the prompt such as adding head turn to the gaze-based cuing. However, if the child is still unable to pick up the

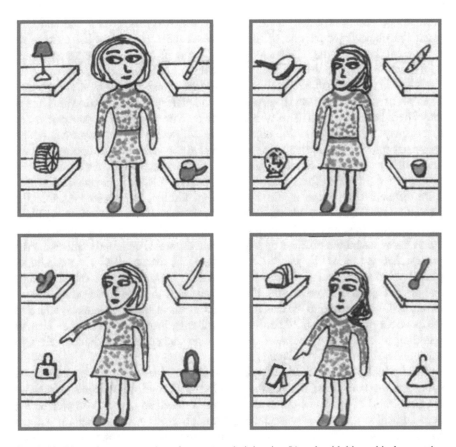

Fig. 5.11 Thematic representation of an avatar administering JA task with hierarchical prompting in a VR-based JA task [4 photos of prompting]

cuing prompt, then the therapist can add a pointing gesture to the previously used prompting cues. For example, the therapist can raise a pointing finger along with gaze orientation and head turn to point towards the target of interest.

Taking inputs from the conventional observation-based studies, researchers such as Jyoti and Lahiri (2019) have designed a VR-based JA task platform for children with autism. Both children with autism and their age-matched typically developing (TD) children took part. For this study, the researchers designed a VR-based room environment with shelves, hanging from the walls on either side of an avatar (a 3D humanoid character) who administered the JA task. Figure 5.11 shows a thematic representation. The shelves displayed virtual objects randomly acquired from a database created from objects selected from the Bank of Standardized Stimuli (BOSS) (Brodeur et al. 2010). The objects used were clock, lamp shade, bowl, etc. The avatar began the task by saying that he or she had lost an object and was trying to find the item in the room and asked the participant to help him or her to find out the object. While the avatar stood inside the VR room, he or she issued various prompting cues and expected the participant to be able to pick up a cue and select the prompted object kept on one of the shelves in the room. Also, the tasks were designed to have varying challenge levels in terms of VR rooms being populated with more objects, thereby increasing the number of options in the JA task.

The avatar was capable of deciding the prompting cue that he or she might use. Thus, at first, the avatar issued a gaze-based prompt by orienting gaze towards one of the objects kept on a shelf. This was followed by a menu-driven response interface that displayed the images of the objects along with radio buttons (representing the response options). The participant was expected to choose one of the options. In case the participant could not select the prompted object correctly, then the avatar moved to a next task in which the avatar walked to another VR room having objects that were different from those in the earlier room. Further, the avatar increased the prompting information by adding head turn to the gaze-based prompting. Again, if the participant was not able to pick up the prompt and did not select the cued object, the avatar repeated the exercise by walking to a different room and demonstrated a prompt that was more informative. For example, the avatar raised a pointed finger (that is pointing gesture) along with head turn and gaze-based cues to point towards one of the objects of interest. Still, if the avatar found that the participant had been unsuccessful in picking up the cue, then an environment-triggered cue was added to the previous cuing prompt. The environment-triggered cue was in the form of sparkling object. This is because children with autism often exhibit interest in shiny and sparkling objects (Coulter 2009).

Results indicated that all the TD participants were able to pick up the gaze-based cuing prompt. In contrast, none of the participants with autism were able to pick up the gaze-based cuing. Some of the participants with autism were able to pick up the head turn along with gaze-based cuing prompt. However, the majority of the participants with autism were successful in picking up the prompting cue comprising of the gaze orientation, head turn, and finger-pointing gesture. Only a small fraction of this target group were incapable of picking up this cue, and subsequently, they were offered the environment-triggered prompting in which the cued object was made to sparkle. Also, the results indicated that multiple exposures could bring in some improvement in the ability of picking up a cuing prompt among the children with autism.

5.5   Summary

In this chapter, I have introduced the reader to some of the design considerations while forming the Virtual Reality (VR)-based scenarios that can be used for different applications. One of the main benefits of using VR from the designer's perspective is the flexibility of design, thereby enabling the designer to present a stimulus to the user based on the experimental paradigm. Also, it enables controlled environments to be presented to the user that can help in the learning of skills by the user. Thus, one of the main ingredients of the VR-based presentation is the audio-visual stimulus that can give a realistic presentation of different social contexts. While VR can be used for various applications, in this chapter, the reader was introduced to the design considerations of user interfaces of VR-based social communication training for children with autism. Additionally, the controllable feature of VR-based stimulus presentation can be achieved by using various techniques, one of which is the State Machine representation. In this chapter, the reader was introduced to such a technique that was used to make the VR-based stimulus adaptive to the performance of the user. Also, the reader was introduced to some of the experimental designs followed by the presentation of the findings of the experimental studies. Similar aspects of experimental design were presented to the reader while using VR-based systems for emotion recognition task and joint attention skill training.

To summarize, we can see that the VR-based skill training platform can hold promise in imparting skill learning in children with autism. Though VR offers a synthetic training world that might be devoid of the subtle niceties of the real world, yet the flexible, controllable, and cost-effective VR-based platform can be potent to offer initial skill training to this target group. Also, experimental studies have shown that such a system has potential to be accepted by the target group. Being affordable, such a training platform can be easily accessed by many while addressing at least some of the core deficits characterizing these children. Thus, it can serve as a complementary tool in the hands of the interventionists working with these children.

References

APA (1994) Diagnostic and statistical manual of mental disorders, 4th edn. American Psychiatric Association, Washington, DC

APA (2000) Diagnostic and statistical manual of mental disorders: DSM-IV-TR. American Psychiatric Association, Washington, DC

Baron-Cohen S, Ring HA, Wheelwright S, Bullmore ET, Brammer MJ, Simmons A, Williams SCR (1999) Social intelligence in the normal and autistic brain: an fMRI study. Eur J Neurosci 11 (6):1891–1898

Bee H, Boyd D (2004) The developing child, 10th edn. Pearson, Boston

Bono MA, Daley T, Sigman M (2004) Relations among joint attention, amount of intervention and language gain in autism. J Autism Dev Disord 34(5):495–505

Booth T (1967) Sequential machines and automata theory. John Wiley and Sons, New York

Brodeur MB, Dionne-Dostie E, Montreuil T, Lepage M (2010) The bank of standardized stimuli (BOSS), a new set of 480 normative photos of objects to be used as visual stimuli in cognitive research. PLoS One 5:e10773

Bruinsma Y, Koegel RL, Koegel LK (2004) Joint attention and children with autism: a review of the literature. Ment Retard Dev Disabil Res Rev 10(3):169–175

Canon PR, Hayes AE, Tipper SP (2009) An electromyographic investigation of the impact of task relevance on facial mimicry. Cognit Emot 23(5):918–929

Carpenter M, Pennington BF, Rogers SJ (2002) Interrelations among social-cognitive skills in young children with autism. J Autism Dev Disord 32(2):91–106

Caruana N, McArthur G, Woolgar A, Brock J (2017) Detecting communicative intent in a computerised test of joint attention. PeerJ 5:e2899. https://doi.org/10.7717/peerj.2899

Caruana N, Ham HS, Brock J, Woolgar A, Kloth N, Palermo R, McArthur G (2018) Joint attention difficulties in autistic adults: an interactive eye-tracking study. Autism 22(4):502–512

Chasson GS, Harris GE, Neely WJ (2007) Cost comparison of early intensive behavioral intervention and special education for children with autism. J Child Fam Stud 16:401–413

Cobb SVG, Nichols S, Ramsey A, Wilson JR (1999) Virtual reality induced symptoms and effects. Presence 8(2):169–186

Constantino JN (2002) The social responsiveness scale. Western Psychological Services, Los Angeles, CA

Coulter RA (2009) Understanding the visual symptoms of individuals with autism spectrum disorder (ASD). Optom Vis Dev 40(3):164–175

Dawson G (2008) Early behavioral intervention, brain plasticity, and the prevention of autism spectrum disorder. Dev Psychopathol 20(3):775–803

Dunn LM, Dunn LM (1997) PPVT-III: Peabody picture vocabulary test, 3rd edn. American Guidance Service, Circle Pines, MN

Eisenbarth H, Alpers GW (2011) Happy mouth and sad eyes: scanning emotional facial expressions. Emotion 11(4):860–865

Ferraioli SJ, Harris SL (2011) Teaching joint attention to children with autism through a sibling-mediated behavioral intervention. Behav Interv 26(4):1921–1962

Ganz ML (2007) The lifetime distribution of the incremental societal costs of autism. Arch Pediatr Adolesc Med 161(4):343–349

Goodwin MS (2008) Enhancing and accelerating the pace of autism research and treatment: the promise of developing innovative technology. Focus Autism Other Dev Disabil 23:125–128

Itti L, Dhavale N, Pighin F (2003) Realistic avatar eye and head animation using a neurobiological model of visual attention. Proc Int Symp Opt Sci Tech 5200:64–78

Jones W, Carr K, Klin A (2008) Absence of preferential looking to the eyes of approaching adults predicts level of social disability in 2-year-old toddlers with autism spectrum disorder. Arch Gen Psychiatry 65(8):946–954

Jonides J, Lewis RL, Nee DE, Lustig CA, Berman MG, Moore KS (2008) The mind and brain of short-term memory. Annu Rev Psychol 59:193–224

Jyoti V, Lahiri U (2019) Virtual reality based joint attention task platform for children with autism. IEEE Trans Learn Technol. https://doi.org/10.1109/TLT.2019.2912371

Lahiri U, Warren Z, Sarkar N (2011) Design of a gaze-sensitive virtual social interactive system for children with autism. IEEE Trans Neural Syst Rehabil Eng 19(4):443–452

Lahiri U, Bekele E, Dohrmann E, Warren Z, Sarkar N (2013) Design of a virtual reality based adaptive response technology for children with autism. IEEE Trans Neural Syst Rehabil Eng 21(1):55–64

Little GE, Bonnar L, Kelly SW, Lohan KS, Rajendran G (2016) Gaze contingent joint attention with an avatar in children with and without ASD. In: 2016 Joint IEEE International Conference on Development and Learning

Lord C, Risi S, Lambrecht L, Cook EH, Leventhal BL, DiLavore PC, Pickles A, Rutter M (2000) The autism diagnostic observation schedule-generic: a standard measure of social and communication deficits associated with the spectrum of autism. J Autism Dev Disord 30(3):205–223

McGee GG, Feldman RS, Morrier MJ (1997) Benchmarks of social treatment for children with autism. J Autism Dev Disord 27:353–364

McIntosh DN, Reichmann-Decker A, Winkielman P, Wilbarger JL (2006) When the social mirror breaks: deficits in automatic, but not voluntary mimicry of emotional facial expressions in autism. Dev Sci 9:295–302

Meindl JN, Cannella-Malone HI (2011) Initiating and responding to joint attention bids in children with autism: a review of the literature. Res Dev Disabil 32(5):1441–1454

Moody EJ, McIntosh DN, Mann LJ, Weisser KR (2007) More than mere mimicry? The influence of emotion on rapid facial reactions to faces. Emotion 7(2):447–457

Mundy P, Sullivan L, Mastergeorge AM (2009) A parallel and distributed processing model of joint attention, social-cognition and autism. Autism Res 2:2–21

NRC (2001) Educating children with autism. National Academy Press, Washington, DC

Paparella T, Goods KS, Freeman S, Kasari C (2011) The emergence of nonverbal joint attention and requesting skills in young children with autism. J Commun Disord 44(6):569–583

Parsons S, Mitchell P (2002) The potential of virtual reality in social skills training for people with autistic spectrum disorders. J Intellect Disabil Res 46:430–443

Pereira AF, Yu C, Smith LB, Shen H (2009) A first-person perspective on a parent-child social interaction during object play. In: Proc. 31st Annual Meeting of Cog. Sc. Society, Amsterdam

Rutherford MD, Towns MT (2008) Scan path differences and similarities during emotion perception in those with and without autism spectrum disorders. J Autism Dev Disord 38:1371–1381

Rutter M, Bailey A, Berument S, Lord C, Pickles A (2003a) Social communication questionnaire. Western Psychological Services, Los Angeles, CA

Rutter M, Le Couteur A, Lord C (2003b) Autism diagnostic interview revised WPS edition manual. Western Psychological Services, Los Angeles, CA

Sigman M, Kasari C (1995) Joint attention across contexts in normal and autistic children. In: Moore C, Dunham PJ, Dunham P (eds) Joint attention: its origins and role in development. Erlbaum, Hillsdale, NJ, p 189

Sigman M, Ruskin E (1999) Continuity and change in the social competence of children with autism, Down syndrome, and developmental delays. Monogr Soc Res Child Dev 64:11–30

Taylor BA, Hoch H (2008) Teaching children with autism to respond to and initiate bids for joint attention. J Appl Behav Anal 41(3):377–391

Trepagnier C, Sebrechts MM, Peterson R (2002) Atypical face gaze in autism. CyberPsychol Behav 5(3):213–217

Whalen C, Schreibman L (2003) Joint attention training for children with autism using behavior modification procedures. J Child Psychol Psychiatry 44:456–468

Chapter 6
Technology-Assisted Skills Training: The Way Forward

6.1 Introduction

So far, the reader has been introduced to some of the core deficit areas characterizing autism and the cascading effects at the later stages of development of these individuals and their families. There has been an increasing consensus that early intervention can help to address many of the core deficits. Thus, the families of such children try their best to offer adequate intervention services to their children. The conventional intervention is mostly observation-based, in which expert clinicians use their knowledge and training to estimate the affective state of the child and in turn tune the intervention paradigm for effective floor-time therapy sessions. The conventional intervention, though powerful, can suffer from few limitations, the most prominent being the restricted availability of trained resources. This becomes a greater challenge given the high prevalence of autism and the necessity of long hours of one-on-one sittings between a clinician with a child while offering individualized services. Such individualization of intervention services is critical since autism is a spectrum disorder in which each child with autism is unique, and thus, the intervention services need to be modulated to cater to the individual needs for effective skill learning. Investigators have been using alternative technology-assisted systems, such as computers augmented with external peripheral devices, that can serve as complementary tools in the hands of the clinicians. In this chapter, I summarize some of the potential strengths of intelligent computing that can make computers be sensitive to one's affective state, be adaptive to one's skill, offer realistic feel through haptics, audio and visual imagery. It is time now to harness these strengths to offer computer-assisted intervention services that can complement the therapists involved in autism intervention.

Faced with such a scenario, investigators have been using alternative techniques that can go hand in hand with the conventional techniques. In other words, the technology-assisted systems can serve as complementary tools in the hands of the clinicians. Throughout the book, the reader has been introduced to the two broad

© Springer Nature Switzerland AG 2020
U. Lahiri, *A Computational View of Autism*,
https://doi.org/10.1007/978-3-030-40237-2_6

types of technology-assisted platforms, namely the computer-assisted and robot-assisted platforms. While robot-assisted platforms have a number of advantages, such as offering 3D embodiment of a facilitator administering a skill training task, controlled skill learning environment with different challenge levels, etc. yet it has some limitations. One of the biggest limitations is the cost of these assistive robots. Though with technological explosion, the price of robots has been decreasing, yet accessibility of robots is still a challenge to countries with developing economy. Thus, investigators have been exploring the use of computers in autism intervention. With the cost of computers going down and availability of graphics cards that can offer rich graphical displays, computer-based specialized applications that can cater to the skill learning of children with autism even in countries with developing economy are becoming feasible.

Given the flexibility in design of specialized applications using computers and ease of interface with external peripheral devices, researchers have been augmenting computer-based systems with various techniques. Thus, computers are no more standalone systems. Instead, the computers can be used to offer audio-visual representations of training scenarios with Virtual Reality (VR), Augmented Reality (AR), and Mixed Reality (MR). Nowadays, interaction with computers has become more realistic since the computers can be interfaced with external peripheral gadgets that can offer a feeling of immersion to the user within the synthetic world. Thus, before being exposed to the real-world scenarios, children with autism can use this computational environment for getting trained in the skills relevant to at least some of the core deficit areas. During the skill learning phase, the child is free to learn by doing, committing mistakes, and practising skills without facing the negative consequences that one can experience while operating in a real-world scenario. With increased penetration of computers even to individual households, the computer-assisted training scenarios can be offered even at the individual homes, thereby allowing the child to learn skill sets while enjoying the comfort of his or her home environment. In other words, computers have become perfect candidates for offering a platform for skill learning for these children and their families.

6.2   Can Computers Offer a Touch of Reality?

Let me devote this section to some of the aspects of computers that might refer to the realistic touch. As mentioned before, with technological progress, computers are now coming with rich graphics and can be easily interfaced with external peripheral devices. This can facilitate users to get a realistic feel of the environment within the simulated world. For example, computers can be coupled with haptic devices that can offer a feeling of touch while interacting with the simulated world presented by the computer. Specifically, the computer can be programmed to generate force feedback using an in-built physics engine when a user collides with an object in the virtual world. The amount of force feedback can be manipulated based on the need. Thus, one can feel the simulated world while performing a task within the environment. Let us consider a training scenario in which one is taught the art of making coffee in the kitchen. In this case, a kitchen environment, having saucer, cups, stove, etc. can be designed in the virtual world. Instead of learning only through visual inspection, such as observing a video, a simulated agent can be used to offer a visual schedule to the learner and walk the learner through the steps used for preparing a cup of coffee. In turn, the learner can learn the art of preparing a cup of coffee by doing it in the virtual world projected by the computer. The learner can first take a pan from the shelf while feeling the touch of the pan, place it on the table while sensing that the table top is supporting the pan with the effects of gravity being added by using a physics engine, etc.

Again, in classroom scenarios (real-life), it often happens that when the teacher understands that a child has acquired mastery in a particular topic having a specific challenge level, the teacher gradually increases the challenge level of the task. Such a scenario can also be programmed in the simulated world. For example, let us consider a social communication skill learning scenario that is offered to a child with autism. Say, a child is in a restaurant scenario that is presented as a synthetic environment to the child. First, the child can be exposed to a restaurant scene that is mostly empty. Thus, the child can walk into the restaurant, order his food at the menu counter, sit at a table, and have food. In case the child faces difficulties in carrying out some of the steps by himself, an artificial agent can be programmed to facilitate the child. If the child is able to do this task by himself without the need to be facilitated, then the computer-based system can offer the child with a restaurant scenario with an increased challenge, such as the restaurant can be projected to be partially full with all the tables as partially occupied. In such a case, the child will be required to exhibit certain social etiquettes before occupying a seat, such as before occupying a seat at one of the tables, the child would be expected to ask permission from the occupants at the table by saying 'Is this seat reserved for someone known to you? Can I take this seat?' If the child is not able to adhere to the social etiquettes, then an artificial agent can be programmed to facilitate the child while taking a seat at one of the tables at the restaurant. In case the child is able to do the task by himself, then the child can be presented a restaurant environment with a task of increased challenge, such as the restaurant environment can be one in which all the tables are completely occupied. In such a case, the child would be expected to stand in a waiting queue and wait for at least a few seats to be empty without causing any tantrums or might decide to get packed food.

Again, computers with VR-based scenarios can allow for safe exploration of the environment by the user, thereby helping the user to learn skills in realistic situations. With technological progress, rich graphics, and increased computing power, graphical display along with depth information can allow for realistic rendering of 3D scenes within the synthetic world. This in turn can offer a touch of reality to the user, thereby contributing to effective skill learning with the possibility of generalization of learnt skills from the simulated world to real-world settings. For example, let us consider a scenario developed to teach the art of navigation while participating in a scavenger hunt exercise. The user might be expected to pick up cues from the environment that can help him in his search for items within the environment. Instead of exposing a child to the real-life world for learning navigation skill, computers can offer a safe (simulated) environment for their exploration. The realistic feel of the synthetic world, coupled with variations, can be motivating for the learner to undergo the skill learning exercise.

Again, another aspect of computers that can offer a sense of reality to the user is through making this synthetic world sensitive to the user's natural response, such as the looking pattern of a user. This is possible because nowadays computers can be seamlessly integrated with cameras and eye tracking devices that can offer a realistic touch to a computer-assisted exercise. While interacting with a social situation, the response in terms of eye gaze shifting is much faster than the other functional modalities such as walking or moving hands. Let me explain this a bit more. Think of a situation in which one can interact with a computer using a mouse or using gaze orientation. Among the two modalities, the gaze orientation can be much faster than the speed at which one can move the mouse and select regions on the computer-based graphical user interface. Again, it is often said that the eyes are the windows to one's mind. In fact, eye movement can be representative of one's mental disposition. Specifically, in a social communication, one's looking pattern varies based on the role of a communicator as a listener or a speaker. Research has indicated a 30–70 rule being used during social communication (Colburn et al. 2000; Argyle and Cook 1976). As per this rule, during social communication, if a social communicator is listening to a partner, then for effective communication, generally, the listener will look at the speaker for about 70% of the time and will look elsewhere for approximately 30% of the time. In contrast, if the communicator is a speaker, then the communicator will look approximately 70% of the time elsewhere and about 30% of the time towards the listener to ensure whether the listener is listening to what the speaker is saying or whether the listener is engaged in social communication. This has been used to define normal gaze from the listener's and the speaker's perspective during social communication. Incorporating such aspects of social communication in the computer-based environment is now possible since computers can be integrated with cameras and eye tracking devices. Let us consider an example that can help explain the touch of reality that eye tracking devices (integrated with computers) can bring to a communication scenario set up using the computing world. Consider an individual is interacting with an intelligent agent designed as a synthetic model in the virtual world. Also, consider three cases in which the individual looks continuously (may be nearly 100% of the time) towards the agent (Case 1) or avoids looking towards the face of the agent (Case 2) or looks about 70% of the time towards the face of the agent (Case 3) while listening to what the agent is telling. Case 1 can be inferred as sticky attention. In such a case if the artificial agent is sensitive to the user's looking pattern, it can be programmed to say

> You have not made be comfortable while I was speaking to you. May be try looking somewhere else, sometimes

This is similar to that what an interventionist might say to a child with autism during intervention. Again, if the individual tends to avoid the eyes of the speaker (agent in this case) (Case 2) that is generally the situation for children with autism, then the agent can be programmed to say

You have not made me comfortable while I was speaking to you. Were you interested in what I was telling you?

Again, if the individual demonstrated normal gaze while listening to the speaker (i.e. the agent) (Case 3), then the agent can be programmed to say

You have made me comfortable while I was speaking to you. It seemed that you were interested in what I was narrating to you.

This can lend a realistic feel to the individual, thereby making the interaction seem natural.

6.3 Affective Computing

Added to the attention-related cues, the ability of a social partner to detect and respond to the affective cues is often crucial for effective social communication. Both performance and affect-related components are important ingredients of social communication. In many cases, the children with autism are capable of offering correct performance in terms of objective task measures. However, these children often face milestones in the affective component of the social communication that in turn can be closely tied to their functional social impairment.

Thus, how about computers be endowed with the power to be able to pick up subtle cues indicative of the affective state of a social communicator (say a child with autism) followed by offering an intelligent response? This can be a way to foster effective social communication skill learning, thereby engaging the child in the social task coupled with a high degree of individualization. This is closely related to the term affective computing that refers to considering the affective information in the human–computer interaction (Picard 1997).

While considering the topic of estimating one's affective response, the question that comes to my mind is 'How to operationalize the Affective State?' Although research on affective computing categorizes one's physiological signal information into basic emotions, consensus on the set of basic emotions is still lacking (Cowie et al. 2001). Thus, one needs to make practical choices while considering the target affective state that can be specific to a particular application. Researchers have often used anxiety as a target affective state. This is because of two main reasons. First of all, human–machine interaction tasks can be modified by an element of anxiety of the actor and this can be closely related with task performance (Brown et al. 1997). The second reason for choosing anxiety while working with children with autism is that anxiety is commonly seen in children with autism that in turn can help to explain the difficulties experienced by these children (Gillott et al. 2001). Again, two other important dimensions can be engagement and liking. The engagement can be considered as 'sustained attention to an activity or person' (NRC 2001) and is thought to be one of the main ingredients that can contribute to achieving substantial gains in academics and social communication domains (Ruble and Robson 2006). Again, if playful activities are developed using computers, then this can offer an avenue to a child with autism to have an enjoyable experience and opportunity to learn along with a motivation to carry out prolonged interaction with other communicators. This is essential since these children often demonstrate a tendency to be withdrawn (Papert 1993).

Research has shown that apart from only exploring one's looking pattern while interacting with a computer, investigating one's physiological signals can lend an eye to the affective state of an individual. It is true that one's facial expressions can convey valuable information on the affective state of an individual during a social task. However, children with autism possess milestones in making explicit expression of their affective states. This can be connected with the communication vulnerabilities that they experience. Thus, tapping into the subtle physiological manifestations of one's affective state can be another alternative. The physiological signals can be evoked involuntarily and controlled by the autonomic nervous system activation. Also, this can offer an undiluted measure of one's affective state since mostly the physiological signals are not susceptible to changes due to communication vulnerabilities characterizing autism. Additionally, physiological signals, though invisible to the naked eye, can be easily picked up and decoded by the computer, thereby offering meaningful inferences on one's affective states. By physiological signals, I refer to the gaze or peripheral physiology. For example, the gaze-related physiology can be in terms of pupillary dilation, blink rate, etc. The peripheral physiology can be in terms of heart rate (computed from electrocardiogram), tonic and phasic activation (evaluated from electrodermal activation), skin temperature, electromyogram activity, etc.

Different researchers have tapped one's physiological signals as indicative of the emotions experienced by an individual. For example, let us consider the work by Picard (2003) in which the researcher refers to the use of different physiological signals for estimating the emotions experienced by an individual. She has used the term 'wearable computer'. In this, she refers to the work of her team offering skin-mounted sensors to recognize one's emotions over an extended duration. The sensors used were meant to record electromyogram, skin conductance, blood volume pulse, and respiration (Picard et al. 2001). All these signals were fed to a classifier and the emotions were detected with an accuracy of more than 81%. In other words, one can say that variations in physiological signals can be representative of varying emotions experienced by an individual.

Again, there are other research studies in which researchers have used physiological signals to tap into the affective state of an individual to develop Virtual Reality (VR)-based social communication training scenarios for children with autism. For example, let us consider the work by Kuriakose and Lahiri (2017). Here the researchers have exposed children with autism to VR-based social communication scenarios that offered various challenges to the participants while teaching various social etiquettes that one can be expected to adhere to in social situations. Such as while visiting a park with see-saws, it might so happen that there are two see-saws. One see-saw is totally empty on both the sides and the other see-saw is partially empty. Now, given the option of using a see-saw, a child with autism might choose the empty see-saw possibly because of his preference to have minimal social interaction with other communicators. In such a case, a virtual facilitator might suggest the participant to choose the partially full see-saw, since the occupant on the see-saw is waiting for someone else to join him or her for playing with the see-saw. However, if the participant selected the partially full see-saw and went to occupy it, then the virtual facilitator might prompt the participant to interact with the occupant at the see-saw by asking him or her whether he or she is expecting any of his or her known acquaintances to join him or her to play with the see-saw. In such social situations, it is quite obvious that the participant might become anxious that might deter him or her to acquire new skills. In such a case, the VR-based system needs to sense the anxiety state of the individual. Here the researchers have used Pulse Plethysmogram (PPG), Skin Temperature (SKT), and Electrodermal Activity (EDA) sensors to extract information on pulse rate, skin temperature, and mean tonic activation, respectively. All of these signals were fed to a fuzzy logic-based Intelligent Anxiety Predictor to estimate the anxiety level that a participant is experiencing while interacting with the VR-based social communication tasks. Thus, if the predicted anxiety was high, then the VR-based system utilized an Adaptive Response Technology to reduce the task challenge level with the hope that the participant will experience lesser anxiety. When the VR-based system could understand that the participant was having reduced anxiety (as predicted from the physiological signals), the VR-based system increased the task challenge level by offering a task of increased difficulty. This has been referred to as an anxiety sensitive system. This system looked at both the anxiety (predicted from the physiological indicators) and the task performance of an individual. The idea was to promote skill learning by the participant while ensuring the comfort of the participant. Then only this can foster effective skill learning. In order to carry out comparative analysis with the other types of response technology, namely one that can be adapted only to one's task performance irrespective of the anxiety state of an individual, the researchers designed a performance sensitive system. The results of the study indicated an increased ability of the anxiety sensitive system to foster improved skill learning compared with that of a performance sensitive system.

The researchers have also been using other modalities, such as gaze-related measures while imparting skill learning for individuals with autism. For example, researchers such as Lahiri et al. (2013) have tapped into one's looking pattern and gaze-related physiology to predict the engagement level of an individual while interacting with a VR-based communication scenario. Specifically, the researchers have used eye tracker to measure one's fixation duration on different regions of interest of the screen along with physiological indices, such as pupil diameter and blink rate. For the purpose of carrying out comparative study, the researchers designed two systems, namely engagement sensitive system and performance sensitive system. In the case of an engagement sensitive system, the manner in which different tasks of varying challenges were offered depended on the cumulative effect of the engagement level (predicted from the eye gaze) and the task performance in an individualized manner. In contrast, the performance sensitive system was made adaptive only to the participant's performance in the VR-based task. The VR-based task was one in which a user could interact with virtual peers projected as virtual characters. Each task had a task presentation phase followed by a back-and-forth communication phase. In the task presentation phase, a virtual character narrated his or her personal experience of participating in a social situation while context-relevant background appeared in the VR scene. In the back-and-forth communication phase, the participant was expected to interact with the virtual character while extracting a piece of information that can be benign, projected contingent, and sensitive in nature that in turn decided the challenge level of the task. The benign information was that related to the context that was narrated by the virtual character during the task presentation phase. A projected contingent information was related to some topic that has not been directly addressed during the task presentation phase, but can be an extension of the topic that was narrated. Again, a sensitive information was one that was related to one's personal feeling. Results of a study carried out with individuals with autism indicated that both the task performance and looking pattern of the participants improved while interacting with the engagement sensitive system as compared to that with the performance sensitive system. Improvement in task performance was measured in terms of the ability of the participants to interact with tasks of increased challenge. Again, improvement in looking pattern was measured in terms of greater fixation towards the face region of the virtual character during social communication. Reduced fixation towards the face of a social communicator along with the tendency to avoid social stimuli (such as faces) is one of the core deficits of the individuals with autism. Improvement in fixation towards the face region of a partner during social communication can be a critical component towards achieving a lucid social communication.

6.4 So, What Next?

To summarize, we can say that computational intelligence can be harnessed to build training platforms that can offer individualized skill training to children with autism. Again, individuals with autism might possess different shades of deficits causing them to be unique that can impose challenges to intervention in terms of individualization of services. Also, there is evidence that in spite of the deficits, individuals with autism have excelled at later stages and there are business establishments that aspire to have these individuals as employees to make use of the attributes in which these individuals can outperform their typically developing counterparts. With increased awareness, children with autism are now in a position to avail early intervention in which many of the core deficits can be addressed. Also, with the intrusion of technology in the life of the common man and individuals becoming computer-savvy, such specialized services can now reach the doorstep and families of these children can easily gain access to these services.

Apart from addressing the skill deficits while harnessing the power of technology, the big question that lies in front of us is, 'Are we trying to understand the strength areas of these children?' Then only we can hone or sharpen their strengths and help them excel in their lives. How about we all join hands and give these individuals a safe place to grow, pursue their dreams, gain success in different walks of life, and co-exist in a meaningful way? I think that those days are not far away.

References

Argyle M, Cook M (1976) Gaze and mutual gaze. Cambridge University Press, Cambridge, MA

Brown RM, Hall LR, Holtzer R, Brown SL, Brown NL (1997) Gender and video game performance. Sex Roles 36:793–812

Colburn A, Drucker S, Cohen M (2000) The role of eye-gaze in avatar-mediated conversational interfaces. In: SIGGRAPH Sketches and Applications, New Orleans, LA

Cowie R, Douglas-Cowie E, Tsapatsoulis N, Votsis G, Kollias S, Fellenz W, Taylor JG (2001) Emotion recognition in human-computer interaction. IEEE Signal Process Mag 18(1):32–80

Gillott A, Furniss F, Walter A (2001) Anxiety in high-functioning children with autism. Autism 5 (3):277–286

Kuriakose S, Lahiri U (2017) Design of a physiology-sensitive VR-based social communication platform for children with autism. IEEE Trans Neural Syst Rehabil Eng 25(8):1180–1191

Lahiri U, Bekele E, Dohrmann E, Warren Z, Sarkar N (2013) Design of a virtual reality based adaptive response technology for children with autism. IEEE Trans Neural Syst Rehabil Eng 21 (1):55–64

National Research Council (NRC) (2001) Educating children with autism. National Academy Press, Washington, DC

Papert S (1993) Mindstorms: children, computers, and powerful ideas, 2nd edn. Basic Books, New York

Picard RW (1997) Affective computing. MIT Press, Cambridge, MA

Picard R (2003) Affective computing: challenges. Int J Hum Comput Stud 59:55–64

Picard RW, Vyzas E, Healey J (2001) Toward machine emotional intelligence: analysis of affective physiological state. IEEE Trans Pattern Anal Mach Intell 23(10):1175–1191

Ruble LA, Robson DM (2006) Individual and environmental determinants of engagement in autism. J Autism Dev Dis 37(8):1457–1468

Printed in the United States
by Baker & Taylor Publisher Services